THE NEW UPDATED DIABETIC GASTROPARESIS DIET COOKBOOK

Easy-to-Follow Recipes to Relieve Symptoms, Prevent Complications, Eliminate Abdominal Pain, Lose Weight, and Stabilize Blood Sugar

Steve Bryant, MD, RD

Copyright Page

Copyright © 2024 Steve Bryant, MD, RD

All rights reserved. No part of this publication may be reproduced, distributed, or transmitted in any form or by any means, including photocopying, recording, or other electronic or mechanical methods, without the prior written permission of the publisher, except in the case of brief quotation embodied in critical reviews and certain other non-commercial uses permitted by copyright law.

Table of Contents

Copyright Page 2

Table of Contents 3

Introduction 1

Chapter 1: Definition and Overview of Gastroparesis 6

    The Most Common Causes of Gastroparesis .. 12

Chapter 2: Understanding Gastroparesis 17

    Symptoms of Gastroparesis 22

Chapter 3: Diagnosing Gastroparesis 28

    Gastroparesis Complications 30

Chapter 4: Gastroparesis Treatment 33

    Gastroparesis Medication 36

Chapter 5: Gastroparesis Foods That Are Suitable for You 40

Avoid These Foods if You Have Gastroparesis. 44

Chapter 6: Gastroparesis Diet Recipes 47

Chicken & Dumpling Soup 47

Chicken Dumplings 50

Fennel & Rice Porridge 52

Ginger Coconut Soup 53

Kitchari 55

Angel Hair Pasta with Shrimp 58

Poached Chicken Pot au Feu 59

Egyptian Yellow Lentil Soup 63

Salmon Pasta Casserole 66

Salmon Quiche 68

Oatmeal 71

The Perfect Hard-Boiled Egg 72

Basic Mustard Vinaigrette 74

Easy Vinaigrette Dressing 75

Basil Pesto 77

Simple Baked Apples 78

Broiled Cod With Puttanesca Sauce 80

Quinoa Bowl With Tahini & Kale 82

Soy Poached Chicken 84

Greek Yogurt Fettuccine Alfredo 86

Poached Salmon With Tarragon Vinaigrette .. 87

Winter Squash Risotto 90

Thai-Style Sweet Potato Curry 93

Simmered Chicken With Daikon Radish 96

Cucumber, Yogurt & Wheat Berry Soup 98

Green Split Pea Soup 100

Chicken With Ginger Broth 102

Egg Noodles in Broth 105

Tarragon & Lemon Chicken Soup With Orzo 106

Matzo Ball Soup 108

Gingery Carrot & Lentil Soup 112

Hoppin' John 115

Cabbage Miso Soup 118

Fall Vegetable Soup With Spicy Gremolata .. 119

Clear Pumpkin Soup 122

Curried Coconut Carrot Soup 124

Wonton Soup With Shiitake Mushrooms 126

Summer Borscht 128

Pumpkin Miso Soup 130

Roasted Garlic Soup 133

Quick Posole 135

Turmeric Dal 138

Broccoli & Almond Soup 140

Cold Roasted Red Pepper Soup 143

Spanish Garlic Soup 145

Fish Sticks With Lemon Mayo 147

Easy White Rice 150

Vegan Hot Chocolate 151

Spicy Turkey Posole 153

Banana Coconut Smoothie 156

Ginger Tea 157

Italian Wedding Soup 158

Peach of a Carrot Zucchini Smoothie 160

Creamy Cashew & Pineapple Green Smoothie 162

Cocoa Cherry Protein Shake 164

Mixed Berry Smoothie 165

Banana Oat Smoothie 166

Chocolate Avocado Smoothie 168

Tropical Protein Smoothie 169

High Protein Blueberry Smoothie 170

Tahini Shake 171

Cold Beet Soup with Honeyed Ricotta 173

Lavender Lemonade 175

Sweet Potato Hummus 176

Roasted Cauliflower Steaks With Sunflower Seed Pesto 178

Peach of a Carrot Zucchini Smoothie 181

Spinach Saag 182

Miso Polenta 184

Tropical Protein Smoothie 186

Vegan Pho 187

Apple Pie Smoothie 189

Chicken & Rice Congee 191

Bananas En Papillote 194

Peanut Butter & Banana Smoothie 195

Poultry Bone Stock 196

Banana Pudding 199

Chicken With Ginger Broth 201

Chicken & Noodles in Coconut Lime Broth . 204

Basic Miso Soup 207

Chicken & Rice Soup 208

Yogurt Marinade 210

Pumpkin Miso Soup 211

Gingersnap Peach Crunch 214

Do Less Day Marinated Roasted Wild Salmon 216

Pear & Peach Sorbet 218

New Breakfast Smoothie (Kefir Berry Protein Smoothie) 219

Protein Powered Onion Soup Dip 220

Low-fat Lemon Buttermilk Tea Bread 222

Frozen Banana Peanut Butter Chocolate Chip Milkshake 224

Squash Herb Bread 225

Spring Pea & Lettuce Soup 227

Impromptu Sweet Potato and Butternut Squash Soup 229

Impromptu Carrot Ginger Soup 231

Baked Potato Tuna Salad 232

Quickie Salmon and Corn Chowder 236

Melon Green Smoothie 237

Choc Dream Smoothie 238

Berry Blast Smoothie 239

Easy Green Smoothie 240

Chapter 7: Final Thought 243

Dietary Advice 245

Nutritional Recommendation 250

Introduction

Gastroparesis is a medical condition characterized by impaired stomach motility, resulting in delayed emptying of gastric contents into the small intestine. This disorder typically arises from nerve damage affecting the intricate network responsible for regulating gastrointestinal movement. Specifically, the vagus nerve, a crucial component of this system, orchestrates the rhythmic contractions of the stomach and intestines to facilitate the smooth passage of food.

The prevalence of gastroparesis is notably high among individuals with long-standing diabetes, particularly those with type 1 diabetes. Research indicates that up to 40 to 50 percent of individuals with type 1 diabetes who have had the condition for more than two decades may develop gastroparesis. Similarly, approximately 30 to 40 percent of individuals with type 2 diabetes in the same duration bracket may also experience gastroparesis.

When the vagus nerve sustains injury or dysfunction, often due to prolonged exposure to elevated blood glucose levels in diabetes, the coordination of gastrointestinal muscle contractions is disrupted. Consequently, the stomach and intestines fail to contract and relax adequately, leading to sluggish or halted movement of food through the digestive tract.

In diabetes, persistent hyperglycemia induces biochemical alterations in nerve function and damages the blood vessels that supply oxygen and nutrients to the nerves. These changes contribute to the deterioration of nerve health, including the vagus nerve, exacerbating the impairment in gastrointestinal motility observed in gastroparesis.

Furthermore, gastroparesis can also arise as a complication of other chronic illnesses, such as lupus, where autoimmune processes may target the nerves or muscles of the digestive system, disrupting their function. Similarly, certain medications and surgical procedures involving the stomach or associated structures can predispose individuals to gastroparesis by interfering with normal gastrointestinal motility.

In essence, gastroparesis represents a complex interplay of physiological and pathological factors, with nerve injury and dysfunction standing at the forefront of its etiology. Understanding these risk factors and their implications is essential for effective management and preventive strategies, particularly in populations vulnerable to gastroparesis development. By addressing the underlying causes and promoting optimal glycemic control in diabetes and mitigating other contributing factors, healthcare professionals can strive to alleviate symptoms and improve outcomes for individuals affected by gastroparesis.

Chapter 1: Definition and Overview of Gastroparesis

Gastroparesis is a chronic and often debilitating medical condition characterized by delayed emptying of the stomach contents into the small intestine, leading to a range of distressing symptoms and complications. The term "gastroparesis" is derived from the Greek words "gastro" (meaning stomach) and "paresis" (meaning partial paralysis), reflecting the underlying dysfunction of the stomach muscles responsible for propelling food along the digestive tract.

In a healthy digestive system, the stomach contracts rhythmically to break down food into smaller particles and mix it with digestive juices before gradually releasing it into the small intestine for further processing and absorption of nutrients. However, in individuals with gastroparesis, this coordinated movement of the stomach muscles is impaired, resulting in slowed or stalled gastric emptying.

The causes of gastroparesis can vary, but the most common underlying factor is damage or dysfunction of the vagus nerve, which plays a crucial role in regulating the muscles of the digestive tract. This damage can occur due to several factors, including diabetes mellitus, which is the leading cause of gastroparesis in the United

States. Other potential causes include neurological disorders, such as Parkinson's disease or multiple sclerosis, as well as surgery on the stomach or esophagus.

The hallmark symptoms of gastroparesis typically include:

- Persistent nausea and vomiting

- Feelings of fullness or bloating after eating even small amounts of food

- Abdominal pain or discomfort

- Acid reflux or heartburn

- Lack of appetite and unintended weight loss

These symptoms can vary in severity and may worsen after consuming certain types of foods or during periods of stress. Gastroparesis can significantly impact an individual's quality of life, leading to nutritional deficiencies, dehydration, and emotional distress.

Diagnosis of gastroparesis often involves a combination of medical history assessment, physical examination, and specialized tests, such as gastric emptying scintigraphy or gastric manometry, to evaluate the function of the stomach muscles and the rate of gastric emptying.

While there is currently no cure for gastroparesis, treatment strategies focus on alleviating symptoms, improving gastric emptying, and preventing complications. This may involve dietary modifications, such as consuming smaller, more frequent meals and avoiding high-fiber or fatty foods that can exacerbate symptoms. Medications to stimulate stomach contractions or manage symptoms like nausea and vomiting may also be prescribed. In severe cases, surgical interventions such as gastric electrical stimulation or pyloroplasty may be considered.

In recent years, there has been growing recognition of gastroparesis as a significant health concern, prompting increased research efforts aimed at better understanding its underlying mechanisms and developing more effective treatment approaches. Despite the challenges posed by this condition, advances in medical science offer hope for improved outcomes and quality of life for individuals living with gastroparesis.

As we delve deeper into the complexities of gastroparesis, it becomes evident that raising awareness, enhancing medical care, and fostering support networks are essential in addressing the needs of those affected by this condition. Through greater understanding and collaboration, we can strive to improve the lives of individuals living with gastroparesis and pave the way for a brighter future.

The Most Common Causes of Gastroparesis

1. Diabetes mellitus, a chronic metabolic disorder characterized by elevated blood sugar levels, stands as a prominent risk factor for the development of gastroparesis. The prolonged exposure to high glucose levels can lead to damage to the vagus nerve, impeding its regulatory function over stomach contractions and subsequently causing delayed gastric emptying.

2. Various syndromes instigated by viral infections present another avenue through which gastroparesis may manifest. Viruses can induce inflammatory responses and damage to the nerves and muscles of the gastrointestinal tract,

disrupting the normal motility of the stomach and contributing to the onset of gastroparesis.

3. Anorexia nervosa, classified as an eating disorder characterized by extreme calorie restriction and an obsessive fear of gaining weight, emerges as another risk factor for gastroparesis. Chronic malnutrition associated with anorexia nervosa can compromise stomach function and impede gastric emptying, exacerbating symptoms of gastroparesis.

4. Surgical interventions targeting the vagus nerve or the stomach itself pose potential risks for the development of gastroparesis as a complication. Procedures such as gastric bypass or surgeries

involving the esophagus may alter the anatomical structures or disrupt nerve pathways, thereby affecting gastric motility and leading to delayed gastric emptying.

5. Certain medications, notably anticholinergics and opioids, are implicated in the pathogenesis of gastroparesis. Anticholinergic drugs can interfere with the signaling pathways responsible for stomach contractions, while opioids, known for their analgesic properties, can slow intestinal contractions, including those of the stomach, contributing to delayed gastric emptying.

6. Although relatively rare, gastroesophageal reflux disease (GERD) can also serve as a risk

factor for gastroparesis. The chronic regurgitation of stomach acid into the esophagus characteristic of GERD can lead to inflammation and damage to the esophageal lining, potentially affecting the function of the nearby stomach and exacerbating symptoms of gastroparesis.

7. Certain medical conditions such as amyloidosis and scleroderma, both examples of smooth muscle diseases, can predispose individuals to gastroparesis. These conditions involve abnormalities in the structure and function of smooth muscle tissues, including those of the gastrointestinal tract, leading to impaired motility and gastric emptying.

8. Disorders of the nervous system, including migraines and Parkinson's disease, represent additional risk factors for the development of gastroparesis. These neurological conditions can disrupt the communication between the brain and the gastrointestinal tract, altering stomach motility and contributing to delayed gastric emptying.

9. Metabolic disorders such as hypothyroidism, characterized by insufficient thyroid hormone production, can also increase the risk of gastroparesis. Metabolic imbalances associated with hypothyroidism and other metabolic disorders can affect various bodily functions, including gastrointestinal motility, potentially leading to delayed gastric emptying and symptoms of gastroparesis.

Chapter 2: Understanding Gastroparesis

Gastroparesis, also known as delayed gastric emptying, presents a challenging landscape within the realm of digestive system disorders. This condition manifests when food remains in the stomach for an extended period, a departure from the normal digestive process. Underpinning this delay is the impairment of nerves crucial for food propulsion through the digestive tract, resulting in dysfunctional muscle activity and a backlog of undigested food within the stomach. Chief among the contributing factors to this condition is diabetes mellitus, a prevalent instigator known for its detrimental impact on nerve health and glycemic control.

Individuals grappling with gastroparesis often bear the burden of vagus nerve injury. This injury impedes the timely transmission of signals necessary for food breakdown, ultimately obstructing nerve activity and hampering digestion. Despite its profound implications, gastroparesis frequently eludes detection and is prone to misdiagnosis, particularly in individuals with chronically elevated blood glucose levels. Prolonged hyperglycemia inflicts pervasive nerve damage throughout the body, exacerbating the risk of developing gastroparesis.

Moreover, sustained elevation of blood glucose levels inflicts harm upon the arteries responsible for transporting vital nutrients and oxygen to the body's neural and organ systems. The collateral damage extends to critical conduits like the vagus nerve and the digestive tract, both integral to the genesis of gastroparesis. As a progressive condition, gastroparesis stealthily unfolds with symptoms such as recurrent heartburn and nausea, often ensnaring individuals in its grip unbeknownst to them.

The ramifications of gastroparesis extend beyond its initial manifestation, significantly complicating glucose management in individuals with diabetes. The delayed digestion exacerbates the challenge of regulating blood glucose levels, precipitating fluctuations that defy prediction. Hence, it is imperative for individuals experiencing irregular glucose levels and associated symptoms to communicate openly with their healthcare providers, facilitating comprehensive management strategies.

Enduring the throes of gastroparesis is an arduous journey fraught with dietary restrictions and the relentless pursuit of blood sugar stability amidst persistent nausea and discomfort. This chronic illness exacts a toll not only on the physical well-being of affected individuals but also on their emotional resilience. The daily struggle against symptoms often leaves individuals grappling with frustration and despondency.

Navigating dietary choices becomes paramount for those contending with gastroparesis, necessitating the avoidance of high-fiber and high-fat meals notorious for prolonging digestion. Embracing dietary modifications involves steering clear of certain foods such as uncooked items, rich dairy products, carbonated beverages, high-fiber fruits, and cruciferous vegetables like broccoli. Additionally, healthcare providers recommend consuming smaller, more frequent meals throughout the day, with a preference for blended foods if necessary. Adequate hydration also assumes critical importance, especially in instances where vomiting occurs, to prevent dehydration and mitigate symptoms.

In essence, understanding the multifaceted nature of gastroparesis and its intertwined relationship with diabetes illuminates the path towards effective management and improved quality of life for those impacted by this intricate condition. By fostering a holistic approach encompassing dietary adjustments, vigilant glucose monitoring, and empathetic support, individuals grappling with gastroparesis can traverse the challenges ahead with resilience and hope.

Symptoms of Gastroparesis

Symptoms associated with gastroparesis can manifest across a spectrum of severity, ranging from mild discomfort to debilitating distress.

These symptoms encompass a wide array of gastrointestinal disturbances, including:

- Bloating and frequent episodes of vomiting, often of undigested food particles.

- Early satiety or a premature sense of fullness shortly after consuming meals, leading to reduced food intake.

- Unintended weight loss, which may occur due to decreased appetite and inadequate nutrient absorption.

- Abdominal discomfort characterized by cramping, pain, or a general feeling of unease.

- Nausea, a persistent sensation of queasiness or the urge to vomit, which can significantly impact daily functioning.

- Heartburn or acid reflux, often accompanied by stomach cramps and discomfort.

- Challenges in maintaining stable blood glucose levels, especially in individuals with diabetes mellitus, due to erratic digestion and absorption of carbohydrates.

- Fluctuations in appetite, ranging from a complete lack of interest in food to intermittent cravings or aversions.

While gastroparesis can occasionally manifest as a transient symptom associated with acute illness or medical procedures, it more commonly presents as a chronic, long-term condition. Certain medical interventions, such as bariatric surgery or other abdominal surgeries, can disrupt normal digestive processes and precipitate the development of gastroparesis.

Dietary habits play a pivotal role in managing gastroparesis symptoms, with modifications often serving as the cornerstone of treatment. Tailoring the intake of lipids and dietary fiber can exert a significant influence on the severity and frequency of symptoms experienced. Therefore, individuals with gastroparesis are advised to make strategic adjustments to their dietary patterns, emphasizing easily digestible foods while minimizing those that are high in fat or fiber.

Furthermore, dietary modifications should be individualized to accommodate each person's unique needs and symptomatology. Collaborating closely with healthcare providers, including dietitians and gastroenterologists, can help individuals with gastroparesis develop personalized dietary plans that optimize nutritional intake while mitigating symptom exacerbations.

In summary, gastroparesis presents a diverse array of symptoms that can profoundly impact an individual's quality of life. Understanding the multifaceted nature of this condition, including its potential triggers and the role of dietary management, is essential for effective symptom control and overall well-being. Through a comprehensive approach that integrates medical management, lifestyle modifications, and dietary adjustments, individuals with gastroparesis can strive to achieve symptom relief and enhance their overall health outcomes.

Chapter 3: Diagnosing Gastroparesis

Prior to diagnosing diabetic gastroparesis, your physician will meticulously examine several variables. They will thoroughly review your medical history and symptoms, in addition to conducting a comprehensive physical examination to identify potential indicators of gastroparesis. These signs may encompass:

- Sensitivity or discomfort in the abdominal region

- Symptoms of dehydration

- Evidence of malnutrition

Furthermore, your doctor may opt to perform blood or urine tests to exclude any underlying issues related to gastroparesis. Imaging tests might also be employed to detect any obstructions within the abdominal cavity. Additionally, procedures such as esophagogastroduodenoscopy or gastric emptying scintigraphy may be conducted.

Esophagogastroduodenoscopy serves the dual purpose of ruling out infections and identifying any food residue that may have accumulated within the stomach. Gastric emptying scintigraphy, on the other hand, is a diagnostic technique employed to assess the rate of gastric emptying, considered the gold standard in diagnosing gastroparesis. Through these meticulous assessments and diagnostic procedures, healthcare providers aim to accurately diagnose and effectively manage diabetic gastroparesis, facilitating optimal patient care and outcomes.

Gastroparesis Complications

Prolonged retention of food within the stomach can lead to various complications, including bacterial overgrowth resulting from fermentation of the undigested food. Additionally, food particles may aggregate and solidify into concretions known as bezoars, posing a risk of inducing symptoms such as nausea, vomiting, and stomach obstruction. Bezoars, if left untreated, can impede the passage of food into the small intestine, exacerbating the gastrointestinal distress.

Moreover, the presence of gastroparesis can exacerbate the management of diabetes by complicating blood glucose control. When delayed stomach emptying causes a backlog of food entering the small intestine for absorption, it can trigger spikes in blood glucose levels. The erratic emptying patterns characteristic of gastroparesis further compound the challenge of maintaining stable blood sugar levels, as individuals may experience unpredictable fluctuations that are difficult to regulate through conventional means. This instability in blood glucose regulation not only undermines metabolic control but also increases the risk of diabetic complications and necessitates vigilant monitoring and adjustment of treatment strategies. Hence, gastroparesis presents a multifaceted challenge in the management of diabetes, requiring a comprehensive approach to optimize therapeutic outcomes and mitigate associated risks.

Chapter 4: Gastroparesis Treatment

Your physician will likely make adjustments to your insulin regimen as deemed necessary for managing your condition effectively. These adjustments may include the following recommendations:

- Altering the frequency or type of insulin you are taking, potentially transitioning to a different formulation that better suits your needs.

- Administering insulin after meals rather than before to better align with your body's natural insulin response to food intake.

- Monitoring your blood glucose levels regularly after meals and administering insulin as required to maintain optimal control.

Furthermore, your healthcare provider may offer more detailed instructions on the timing and dosage of your insulin administration tailored to your individual needs and circumstances.

In cases of severe gastroparesis, your doctor may consider gastric electrical stimulation as a treatment option. This procedure involves the surgical placement of a device in your abdomen, which emits electrical impulses to stimulate the nerves and smooth muscles of your lower stomach. This stimulation aims to alleviate symptoms such as nausea and vomiting, improving overall gastric function.

For individuals with long-term gastroparesis, particularly those experiencing significant difficulties with oral intake, the management approach may involve the use of liquid diets and feeding tubes in extreme circumstances. These interventions ensure adequate nutrition and hydration while bypassing the challenges associated with impaired gastric motility.

It's essential to maintain open communication with your healthcare team regarding your symptoms, treatment preferences, and any concerns you may have. Together, you can work towards developing a comprehensive management plan that addresses your unique needs and optimizes your quality of life despite the challenges posed by gastroparesis.

Gastroparesis Medication

Various medications are utilized in the treatment of gastroparesis. Your healthcare provider may conduct trials with different medications or combinations thereof to ascertain the most effective treatment regimen for you.

Metoclopramide, classified as an antiemetic (commonly known as Reglan), induces muscular spasms in the stomach to facilitate food emptying.

Additionally, it aids in reducing symptoms of nausea and vomiting. Typically administered 20 to 30 minutes before meals and bedtime, metoclopramide may induce side effects such as fatigue, drowsiness, melancholy, anxiety, and difficulties with physical mobility.

Another medication, erythromycin, which is an antibiotic, also accelerates gastric emptying by strengthening contractions that propel food through the stomach. Nausea, vomiting, and stomach cramping may occur as side effects.

Domperidone, another medication under review by the Food and Drug Administration for gastroparesis treatment, functions similarly to cisapride and metoclopramide by enhancing gastric motility. Additionally, domperidone alleviates symptoms of nausea.

Furthermore, there are other medications that may be employed to address gastroparesis symptoms and associated complications. For instance, antiemetics can be beneficial in managing nausea and vomiting, while antibiotics may be prescribed to treat bacterial infections. In cases of bezoars, where there is a concretion of indigestible material in the gastrointestinal tract, medication may be injected via an endoscope to dissolve the bezoar.

The selection of medications and treatment strategies should be tailored to individual patient needs and considerations, with close monitoring for effectiveness and potential adverse effects. Your healthcare provider will work with you to devise a comprehensive treatment plan aimed at managing your gastroparesis symptoms and optimizing your quality of life.

Chapter 5: Gastroparesis Foods That Are Suitable for You

If you are grappling with the challenges of gastroparesis, it becomes paramount to prioritize your nutritional intake, ensuring a delicate balance of essential nutrients while navigating through dietary choices. Embracing a dietary regimen characterized by small, frequent meals emerges as a cornerstone strategy in managing gastroparesis effectively. These meals should ideally be low in fat and easily digestible, fostering minimal strain on the compromised gastrointestinal system.

In crafting a diet tailored to mitigate the symptoms of gastroparesis, emphasis is placed on incorporating foods rich in high-quality proteins, such as eggs and creamy nut butter, which not only provide essential amino acids for bodily functions but also contribute to a prolonged feeling of satiety. Additionally, the inclusion of easily digestible vegetables, such as cooked zucchini, bolsters the nutritional profile of the diet while minimizing the burden on the digestive system.

The texture and consistency of food play a pivotal role in easing the digestive process for individuals with gastroparesis. Opting for foods that are soft, smooth, and effortless to chew and swallow enhances the likelihood of efficient digestion and absorption of nutrients. Hence, a repertoire of easily digestible foods becomes indispensable in crafting meals that are gentle on the stomach yet nutritionally dense.

In navigating the culinary landscape amidst gastroparesis, a curated list of foods emerges as allies in managing symptoms and promoting overall well-being. Smooth or creamy options like peanut butter and eggs offer a palatable and nutrient-rich foundation for meals, providing a blend of essential macronutrients to sustain bodily functions.

Furthermore, bananas, with their naturally soft texture and rich potassium content, emerge as a versatile and easily digestible fruit choice. Similarly, opting for white breads, low-fiber cereals, and low-fat crackers ensures a gentle dietary transition, minimizing the risk of exacerbating gastrointestinal symptoms.

Juices crafted from fruits and vegetables, such as spinach, kale, and carrots, offer a refreshing and nutrient-packed alternative to solid foods, facilitating hydration and nutrient absorption. Incorporating pureed fruits into the dietary repertoire provides a convenient and palatable means of meeting nutritional needs while accommodating the unique challenges posed by gastroparesis.

By embracing a dietary approach centered around easily digestible, nutrient-dense foods, individuals with gastroparesis can optimize their nutritional status, alleviate symptoms, and enhance their overall quality of life. Through mindful dietary choices and a tailored approach to nutrition, navigating the complexities of gastroparesis becomes a more manageable journey towards improved health and well-being.

Avoid These Foods if You Have Gastroparesis.

When grappling with symptoms of gastroparesis, it becomes imperative to be well-versed in dietary choices that can either alleviate or exacerbate your condition. Foods laden with high fat or fiber content should be approached with caution and consumed in moderation. Here's an exhaustive list of items notorious for potentially aggravating gastroparesis symptoms:

- Carbonated beverages, notorious for their potential to cause bloating and discomfort.

- Legumes and beans, including alcohol beans, known to be heavy on the stomach and difficult to digest.

- Corn seeds and nuts, notorious for their fibrous content, which can impede digestion.

- Cruciferous vegetables such as broccoli and cauliflower, which may induce bloating and gas.

- Cheese, particularly high-fat varieties, which can be difficult for the stomach to process.

- Heavy cream, known for its richness and potential to exacerbate symptoms of gastroparesis.

- Excessive oil or butter, which can overwhelm the digestive system and slow down gastric emptying.

Being mindful of these dietary culprits and making informed choices can play a pivotal role in managing gastroparesis symptoms and enhancing overall well-being. It's advisable to consult with a healthcare professional or a registered dietitian to tailor a dietary plan that suits your specific needs and preferences while mitigating the impact of gastroparesis on your daily life.

Chapter 6: Gastroparesis Diet Recipes

Chicken & Dumpling Soup

Ingredients

Soup:

1 teaspoon plus 1 tablespoon olive oil

6 skinless chicken drumsticks (See Chef Tips)

1 medium onion, chopped

4 small celery ribs, cut into ½-inch dice

4 carrots, cut into ½-inch dice

1 bay leaf

Salt and pepper, to taste

6 cups low-sodium chicken broth or water

Dumplings:

1½ cups all-purpose flour

½ cup cornmeal

1 tablespoon baking powder

Salt, to taste

1 cup milk

¾ cup plain Greek yogurt

Dumplings are the ultimate comfort food. Every culture makes them in one form or another; think idly, gnocchi or matzo balls. They are often added to soups and stews to bulk them up.

Preparation

In a heavy-bottomed pot, heat 1 teaspoon of oil over medium-high heat. Brown the chicken in batches. Then remove from pot and set aside.

Add 1 tablespoon of olive oil to the same pot and cook the onions, celery, carrot, and bay leaf. Sprinkle with a generous pinch of salt and sauté for 5-8 minutes or until the onions are translucent.

Add the browned chicken back to the pot with the broth or water. Bring to a boil. Reduce heat and simmer for at least 30 minutes.

Remove chicken from the soup with tongs and using a fork pull the meat from the bone. Return to the soup and discard the bones.

To make the dumplings: In a small bowl mix all the dumpling ingredients until combined.

Bring the soup to a gentle simmer then drop tablespoonfuls of the batter into the soup. They will rise to the top when they are cooked. Simmer for 15 minutes.

Taste for seasonings. Serve.

Chicken Dumplings

Ingredients

1 pound ground chicken

¼ cup soy sauce

1 bunch scallions, minced

5 cloves garlic, minced

1 inch ginger, peeled and minced

30 wonton wrappers

Preparation

In a bowl combined ground chicken, soy sauce, scallions, garlic, and ginger and mix well.

To make each dumpling, place about 2 teaspoons of ground chicken in the center of each wrapper. When ready to shape, brush two of the edges with water. Fold the dry sides onto the wet sides to form a triangle. Press with your fingers to make sure they are closed.

Place the shaped dumplings onto a baking sheet. Once all the filling and wrappers are used, place the dumplings in the freezer until cold and reserve until needed. To cook, boil in broth or water until cooked through, about five minutes.

Fennel & Rice Porridge

Ingredients

2 cups Basmati rice

4 cups low-sodium chicken or vegetable stock

6 cups water

1 medium fennel bulb (about 2 cups) chopped

2 cups frozen peas.

4 eggs, hard boiled, peeled and quartered

¼ cup fennel fronds, chopped (optional)

Preparation

In a large pot, combine rice, chicken stock, water, and fennel. Place the pot on the stove, set to medium heat.

Bring the rice to a simmer and cover. Cook stirring occasionally for about 45 minutes or until the rice has absorbed most of the liquid and looks soupy. Stir in the peas, cook the porridge for a minute to thaw them. Remove from the heat and check for salt.

Serve garnished with wedges of egg, and a sprinkle of fennel fronds.

Ginger Coconut Soup

Ingredients

2 (14-ounce) cans of coconut milk

1¼ cup water

1 to 2 tablespoons ginger, freshly grated

2 medium shallots, peeled and sliced lengthwise

Salt, to taste

¾ pound small new potatoes, or ⅓ cup of long grain white rice

1 cup of 1-inch asparagus sliced pieces

1 cup of broccoli florets

Cilantro or Thai basil, for garnish

Preparation

In a medium stockpot, bring the coconut milk, water, ginger, shallots, salt, and potatoes or rice to a boil.

Reduce heat and simmer until the potatoes are tender or the rice is cooked. Add in the vegetables, cook for 3 to 5 minutes sprinkle with chopped cilantro or Thai basil cook one minute more then serve.

Kitchari

Ingredients

2 tablespoons ghee

3 teaspoons mustard seeds

2 teaspoons cumin seeds or powder

2 teaspoons turmeric

2 teaspoons coriander

2 teaspoons fennel seeds

1 pinch asafoetida (hing) (See Chef Tip)

2 cups yellow split peas, picked through, rinsed and drained

Pinch of salt

7 cups water

1 cup brown basmati rice, rinsed and drained a few times

Cilantro, to garnish (optional)

Preparation

Sauté the mustard seeds in the oil or ghee until they pop. Then, add the cumin, turmeric, coriander, fennel seeds and asafetida, if using. Cook for 1 minute.

Add the split peas and salt. Sauté for 1 to 2 minutes. Add water, bring to boil, then simmer for 30 minutes or until the dal is about ⅓ cooked.

Prepare any preferred vegetables (see Chef Tip). Add rice and these vegetables.

Stir to mix, adding extra water if required. Bring back to a boil, then simmer for 20 minutes or until rice is fully cooked and the water is completely absorbed.

Angel Hair Pasta with Shrimp

Ingredients

1 pound angel hair pasta

3 tablespoons olive oil

2 cloves garlic, minced, about 2 teaspoons

1 teaspoon red pepper flake

12 ounces shrimp, peeled, deveined

1 lemon, juiced, about 2 tablespoons

½ cup basil leaves

Preparation

In a large saucepot, boil 6 quarts of salted water.

While water is coming to a boil, heat a large saute pan with olive oil over medium heat. Saute garlic 1 minute until soft. Add the pepper flakes, cook an additional minute. Remove from heat.

Cook pasta until al dente, following package directions.

Return saute pan to heat. Add shrimp, cook for 2 minutes, stirring occasionally. Add about ¼ cup of the pasta water to the saute pan, stirring.

Add cooked pasta to pot. Season with lemon and add the basil leaves. Cook 30 seconds and toss pasta together and serve.

Poached Chicken Pot au Feu

Ingredients

2 small yellow onions, peeled and cut in half

8 cloves

2 leeks, trimmed and washed well, dark tops reserved

1¾ pounds skinless chicken breast, on the bone

3 medium carrots, scrubbed and cut into 3 equal lengths, then into quarters lengthwise

4 small white turnips, peeled and quartered

1 bay leaf

½ teaspoon black peppercorns

4 to 6 cups water

Sea salt to taste

1⅓ cups of Arborio or other short-grain rice

Fresh parsley, to garnish (optional)

Dijon mustard, for serving (optional)

Preparation

Stud each onion half with two cloves. Cut the white part of the trimmed leeks into three equal lengths, then in half lengthwise. Set aside. Cut the tender parts of the dark tops of the leeks into 3-inch lengths and tie them together with a piece of string.

Put the chicken into a heavy Dutch oven or casserole dish. Cover with water, and bring to a boil over high heat. As soon as the chicken flesh turns white, remove and set aside on a plate. Discard the water.

Rinse the pot. Put in carrots, turnips, bay leaf, peppercorns, bundled leek greens, and onions. Reserve the leek whites. Add enough stock or water to cover the vegetables completely and bring to a boil over a high heat. Cover and turn the heat down to low. Gently simmer the vegetables for 10 minutes.

Add the chicken to the simmering vegetables and top with the reserved leeks. Sprinkle with a little sea salt and cover. Cook at a simmer over very low heat for about 20 minutes. The chicken should be just cooked and the vegetables tender but not mushy. Taste for salt. Add the measured rice directly to the pot, cover, and cook at a low simmer for 15 minutes or until the rice is al dente. Turn off the heat and let the pot sit, covered, for 10 minutes for the rice to steam and the flavors to develop.

To serve, remove the bundled leek greens and discard. Cut the chicken pieces in half. Plate the chicken with half an onion and some carrots, turnips, leek whites, and rice. Spoon stock from the pot over the chicken and vegetables. Serve with Dijon mustard on the side.

Egyptian Yellow Lentil Soup

Ingredients

2 cups dried orange split lentils

8 cups low-sodium broth, as needed, divided

1 medium tomato, chopped

1 thin-skinned potato (like Yukon Gold), cut into a small dice

1 carrot, peeled, cut in a small dice

2 tablespoons olive oil

1 large onion, finely chopped

1 teaspoon ground cumin

1 teaspoon ground turmeric

1 tablespoon fresh parsley or cilantro, chopped

Salt and pepper, to taste

Preparation

In a large saucepan, cover the lentils with 5 cups of stock. Add tomato, potato, carrot, and salt and bring to a boil; reduce heat and simmer for 30 minutes, skimming any foam that forms on top.

Meanwhile, heat oil in a medium pot over medium-high heat. Add the onion and saute for about 2 minutes, then turn the heat to medium-low and cook until golden and caramelized, about 8 minutes. The onions should not be burnt. Stir in the cumin and turmeric, cook 1 minute. Set aside.

Remove the lentil mixture from heat and puree using a hand-held immersion blender or in batches in the regular blender. Add to the onions and spices along with the 3 cups stock. (If you prefer a thicker soup, add less.) Bring soup to a simmer and cook for about 10 minutes, or until thickened. Season to taste with salt and pepper. Serve immediately, topped with Baked Whole Wheat Pita Chips (optional) and parsley or cilantro.

Salmon Pasta Casserole

Ingredients

1 pound whole wheat penne pasta

4 tablespoons butter

½ cup minced onion

2 tablespoons flour

2 cups low-fat milk

2 tablespoons lemon juice

2 tablespoons chopped parsley

Salt to taste

8 ounces canned salmon, drained, flaked, skin and bones removed

1 ½ cups shredded sharp cheddar cheese

Preparation

Cook pasta until just al dente according to package instructions.

To make the sauce, melt the butter in a medium saucepot. Add the onion and sauté until transparent. Add the flour, and stir until combined. Cook for one minute or until the flour turns a light brown.

Slowly stir in the milk. Cook, stirring constantly, until smooth and thick. The mixture should coat the back of a wooden spoon. Add lemon juice, parsley and season with salt.

Spoon pasta into a greased casserole dish. Spread the salmon evenly over the top. Pour on third of the sauce over the pasta and salmon. Sprinkle 3/4 cup of cheese over it. Pour the rest of the sauce over it, and sprinkle with the remaining cheese.

Bake at 375°F for 25 minutes, or until hot and lightly browned.

Salmon Quiche

Ingredients

1 Basic Whole-Wheat Pie Dough (or store-bought crust)

1 (14.75 ounce) can salmon

1 tablespoon lemon juice

1 small onion, minced

2 tablespoons butter

2 tablespoons parsley, chopped

6 eggs, whisked

1 ½ cups milk

¾ cup shredded gruyere

1 teaspoon salt

2 tablespoons chopped chives

Pinch pepper

Preparation

Preheat oven to 400 degrees.

On a clean and floured surface, roll out the pie dough to a ¼ inch thick (if not using a prepared crust) and fit into a pie tin, cutting off the extra dough. Poke a few holes in the crust with a fork. Bake crust in the preheated oven for 5 minutes. Once par-baked, remove it from the oven and let cool slightly. Turn the oven down to 350 °F.

Drain salmon liquid into a cup and reserve. Put salmon in a bowl and remove large bones and skin; flake salmon.

Spread salmon evenly in the baked pie crust; sprinkle with lemon juice.

Cook onion in the butter until translucent; transfer to the pie crust and sprinkle with parsley.

Mix 3 tablespoons of the salmon liquid with eggs, milk and cheese. Stir in the chives. Season with salt and pepper; pour over salmon and onion. Sprinkle with some extra gruyere.

Bake quiche for 45 to 50 minutes, or until firm.

Oatmeal

Ingredients

1 cup rolled oats

2 cups water

Pinch of salt

1 cup apple, chopped (or any fruit of choice)

¼ cup walnuts, chopped (or any other nuts of choice)

¼ cup pumpkin seeds (or any other seeds of choice)

1 tablespoon ground flaxseeds

Preparation

Mix the oats, water, and pinch of salt in a small pot. Cover and cook for 7 to 10 minutes, stirring occasionally. Top with fruit, nuts, seeds, and ground flaxseed. Serve warm

The Perfect Hard-Boiled Egg

Ingredients

4 large eggs

Cold water, to cover

Pinch of salt

Preparation

Take the eggs from the fridge and put them in a pan. Cover them with cold water. Add a pinch of salt. The salt will set any seeping egg white, should an egg crack during boiling.

Bring the eggs to a rolling boil over a medium-high heat. Cover, turn the heat down to medium, and cook for 5 to 6 minutes (see Chef Tips for a soft-boiled egg). This will be enough to set the eggs all the way through.

Take the pan from the heat and place it in the sink. Run cold water over the eggs until the water in the pan is cold. Leave the eggs to sit in the cold water until completely cooled. Store in the fridge to use as needed. They will keep 3 to 4 days.

Basic Mustard Vinaigrette

Ingredients

2 tablespoons Dijon mustard

Salt and freshly ground black pepper, to taste

1 tablespoon white wine vinegar

2 tablespoons extra virgin olive oil

1 tablespoon cold water

1 garlic clove, cut in half, or to taste

Preparation

Spoon the mustard into a large salad bowl, with a pinch of salt and a grind or two of black pepper. Add the vinegar to the mustard and whisk until completely blended and smooth.

Beating continuously, slowly add the oil into the mustard mixture until it is all combined and you have a thick smooth cream. Add half of the water and beat to blend. Taste for sharpness. If it is still too sharp, beat in the rest of the water, or a little more oil, depending on how light you like your dressing. Adjust for salt and it"s ready!

Easy Vinaigrette Dressing

Ingredients

1 tablespoon white wine vinegar

Sea salt and freshly ground black pepper, to taste

Pinch of brown sugar (optional)

3 tablespoons extra virgin olive oil

1 tablespoon water, or to taste

Preparation

In a bowl whisk together the vinegar, salt, pepper, and sugar if using, until the salt has dissolved.

Gradually beat in the olive oil until well blended. Taste for sharpness. If the dressing is too sharp, beat in some water, a little at a time, until the dressing is to your taste.

Basil Pesto

Ingredients

2 to 3 cloves of garlic

¾ cup of pine nuts, toasted until golden and cooled

1 cup grated Parmesan cheese

5 cups sweet basil leaves, washed

Sea salt and pepper, to taste

½ cup extra virgin olive oil

Preparation

In a food processor, pulse the garlic until finely chopped. Add the pine nuts, cheese, basil, salt, and pepper. Process until finely chopped. Keeping the food processor running, add the oil until well blended. Serve immediately, freeze or cover with plastic wrap and chill until ready to use.

Simple Baked Apples

Ingredients

2 to 3 tablespoon sliced almonds, or chopped walnuts

4 tart eating apples, cored

1 tablespoon dried cranberries or raisins

2 to 3 tablespoons maple syrup, or to taste

2 teaspoon butter, or to taste (optional)

1 to 2 tablespoon water

Preparation

Preheat the oven to 375 degrees.

Dry roast the sliced almonds in a heavy pan just until they begin to color. Set aside in a bowl.

Place the apples in a baking dish just big enough to hold them. Stuff them with the dried fruit. Drizzle them with the maple syrup making sure that it gets into the hollowed out core, and then put a nut of butter on top of each one. Add the water to the bottom of the dish.

With a sharp knife, cut a slit in the skin all the way around the waist of each cored apple. This will allow them to expand as they cook.

Broiled Cod With Puttanesca Sauce

Ingredients

12 ounces cod fillet, cut into four equal pieces

Puttanesca Sauce:

4 teaspoons olive oil, divided

½ small onion

1 cup Quick Tomato Sauce

6 green olives, pitted and roughly chopped

6 Kalamata olives, pitted roughly chopped

2 tablespoons capers, drained

1 tablespoon chopped flat leaf parsley

1 tablespoon lemon zest

Salt and pepper, to taste

Preparation

To make the sauce: Heat the olive oil over medium heat. Add the onions and cook until translucent, do not let them brown. Add the Quick Tomato Sauce, olives, and capers. Mix well, reduce heat to medium and simmer for 5 minutes. Stir in the parsley and lemon zest. Cook for 1 minute more. Set aside and keep warm.

Heat the broiler. Lay the cod fillets on a baking sheet lined with foil. Drizzle with olive oil, and sprinkle with salt and pepper. Cook under the broiler for about 8 minutes or until opaque in the center. Top with puttanesca sauce and serve. Pairs well with wilted spinach and Basic Polenta.

Quinoa Bowl With Tahini & Kale

Ingredients

1 teaspoon minced shallot

1 tablespoon olive oil

1 tablespoon tahini

1 tablespoon fresh lemon juice or cider vinegar

Salt, to taste

3 cups finely chopped kale leaves

3 cups cooked Easy Quinoa

¼ cup plain Greek yogurt

½ medium avocado, diced

2 tablespoons chopped olives

2 tablespoon raisins

Fresh pepper, to taste

Chopped cilantro or mint (optional)

Preparation

In a small bowl whisk together the shallot, olive oil, tahini, lemon juice or vinegar, and salt. Add the chopped kale, and stir to mix well. Let sit for at least 10 minutes.

Evenly divide the quinoa between 4 bowls. Top each bowl evenly with the kale, then 1 tablespoon of plain yogurt, diced avocado, chopped olives and raisins. Top with some freshly ground pepper and chopped herbs. Serve at room temperature.

Soy Poached Chicken

Ingredients

2 medium shallots, quartered

1 inch piece of peeled ginger, cut in ¼-inch slices

2 garlic cloves, smashed left whole

2 tablespoons soy sauce

2 inch piece of lemon peel

Juice from one lemon

1 teaspoon sugar

¾ cup water or broth

4 skinless, boneless chicken breasts

Cilantro, for garnish

Preparation

In a wide deep skillet bring the shallots, ginger, garlic, soy sauce, lemon peel, lemon juice, sugar, and water to a boil. Reduce heat and simmer for at least 10 minutes.

Just before serving, add the chicken, cover and cook for 10 minutes. Turn off the heat and continue to steam for 2 to 3 minutes.

Remove the chicken from the pot, and turn the heat up to medium-high. Reduce the sauce for about 3 to 5 minutes or until desired consistency. Pour over chicken and serve with chopped cilantro.

Greek Yogurt Fettuccine Alfredo

Ingredients

1 pound whole-wheat fettuccine

1½ cups whole milk Greek yogurt (see Chef Tips)

1/2 cup grated Parmesan cheese, or to taste (see Chef Tips)

3 tablespoons garlic, minced

¼ cup fresh parsley, chopped

1 teaspoons salt

1 teaspoon ground black pepper

Fresh arugula, to garnish on top (optional)

Preparation

Boil the pasta in salted water for one minute less than package instructions. Reserve 1 cup of the pasta cooking water, then drain the pasta.

In a medium bowl, whisk together yogurt, Parmesan cheese, garlic, and parsley. Slowly whisk in the hot pasta water a little bit at a time. Add the pepper, and taste. Adjust the seasoning with more Parmesan or salt, if needed.

Toss the cooked, hot pasta in the sauce. Serve immediately with extra freshly grated parmesan cheese.

Poached Salmon With Tarragon Vinaigrette

Ingredients

For the Poached Salmon:

1 inch slice of lemon peel

½ teaspoon black peppercorns

1 bay leaf

Salt, to taste

½ small onion (optional)

2 to 4 cups of water

1¼ pounds wild salmon fillet

For the Tarragon Vinaigrette:

2 tablespoons Dijon mustard

Sea salt and freshly ground black pepper, to taste

1 tablespoon white wine vinegar

2 tablespoons extra virgin olive oil

1 tablespoon cold water

3 to 4 good sized sprigs of fresh tarragon, lightly chopped

Preparation

In a wide saute pan with a tight-fitting lid, add the lemon peel, peppercorns, bay leaf, salt, and onion, if using. Add 1-inch of water, then bring to a boil, then cover and simmer for 10 minutes, or until the onion is tender, if using.

Place the salmon skin-side down in the water and cover the pan. Turn off the heat. Let the salmon sit and steam for 8 to 10 minutes, per inch of thickness.

Meanwhile, prepare the vinaigrette. Follow the instructions here.

Remove the salmon and discard the liquid. Drizzle with the tarragon vinaigrette. This dish is good eaten either hot or cold. Serve with Basic Couscous or Simple Roasted Potatoes.

Winter Squash Risotto

Ingredients

1 tablespoon olive oil

1 small yellow onion, chopped

3 pounds kabocha or butternut squash seeded, peeled and cut into a 1-inch dice

4 cups plus 2 cups hot water or low-sodium vegetable stock

2 cups arborio rice

2 tablespoons freshly grated Parmesan cheese, or to taste

2 tablespoons butter, or to taste

1 clove garlic, thinly sliced (if on a bland diet, see Chef Tips)

8 to 10 large, fresh sage leaves, shredded

Sea salt, to taste

Preparation

Heat the olive oil in a Dutch oven over medium heat. Add the onion, sprinkle with salt, and cook until it starts to soften, about 4 to 5 minutes. Add the pumpkin, stir to mix. Cover and sweat over medium heat for 8 minutes, stirring from time to time, or until the pumpkin has started to soften.

Add 4 cups of stock and bring to a boil. Cover the pot, lower the heat, and simmer for 15 minutes, or until the pumpkin is soft. Add the rice, stir to mix, and cook for 15 minutes. The pumpkin will have disintegrated and the rice will be just al dente. Add a little extra stock if it looks very thick. Stir in the Parmesan. Taste for salt.

While the rice is cooking, melt the butter in a small pan or skillet over low heat. Do this slowly for the best results. When the butter has stopped foaming and is clear with nut-brown residue, add the garlic and cook until it is just golden. Remove, turn up the heat a notch, and add the shredded sage leaves. Cook until just crisp, about 2 minutes. Reserve half the leaves.

Stir the butter mixture into the rice. Cover and let sit for 2 minutes. Add a little extra warm stock if the risotto looks dry – it should be a little soupy. Serve immediately sprinkled with the reserved sage leaves and a chunk of Parmesan to grate over the top.

Thai-Style Sweet Potato Curry

Ingredients

3 tablespoons vegetable oil

1 cinnamon stick

4 cloves

4 dried chilies, whole (or to taste, see Chef Tips)

3 garlic cloves, thinly sliced

1 inch fresh ginger, peeled and julienned

4 sweet potatoes, (about 2 pounds) peeled and cut into 1-inch cubes

1 medium onion, finely chopped

1 stalk lemongrass, smashed and tied into a tight bundle

1 (14 ounce) can light coconut milk

1 tablespoon Thai fish sauce (optional)

Salt, to taste (if not using fish sauce)

Juice of ½ a lime

2 to 3 tablespoons fresh cilantro, roughly chopped

Preparation

Heat the oil in a wok or large saute pan over a medium-high heat until it ripples. Add the cinnamon stick, cloves and chilies and cook until the cloves swell and pop and the chilies turn dark, about 1-2 minutes. Add the garlic and fresh ginger and fry, stirring gently until the garlic begins to turn a pale gold color.

Add the sweet potatoes and onions and stir-fry until the onions have softened and begin to brown, about 5-8 minutes. Add the lemongrass, coconut milk, and fish sauce or salt.

Cover, turn down the heat, and simmer for 20 minutes or until the potatoes are tender.

Discard the whole spices and lemongrass. Stir in the lime juice and taste for seasonings. Stir in the chopped cilantro. Turn off the heat and let the curry sit for 1 minute then serve with Easy Brown Rice or Easy White Rice.

Simmered Chicken With Daikon Radish

Ingredients

1 pound chicken drumsticks and thighs, skinned

1 cup sake or dry sherry

¼ cup mirin

2 tablespoons soy sauce

1 teaspoon sugar

1 cup water

1 small daikon radish, about 1 pound, peeled and cut into 1-inch rounds

1 stalk green onion, thinly sliced (optional, see Chef Tips)

1 tablespoon toasted sesame seeds (optional)

Preparation

Bring the chicken, sake, mirin, soy sauce, sugar, and water to a boil in a medium saucepan. Reduce to a simmer and add the daikon. Add water as needed to completely submerge the chicken and daikon. Cover and simmer for 45 minutes to 1 hour, or until the daikon is brown and tender and the chicken is falling off the bone.

Carefully divide the chicken and daikon pieces into serving bowls with a little broth. Top with green onions and some sesame seeds. Eat immediately. Serve with Basic Brown Rice.

Cucumber, Yogurt & Wheat Berry Soup

Ingredients

½ cup wheat berries, preferably soaked overnight

1½ cups chopped, peeled and seeded cucumber

1 bunch spinach leaves, washed

Salt, to taste

1 to 2 cloves of garlic, peeled

1 teaspoon cumin seeds, toasted

3 cups Greek yogurt

½ a lemon, juiced

Fresh mint, chopped

Preparation

Boil the wheat berries until tender and chewy, about 30 minutes if presoaked, or 50 minutes if not. Drain and set aside to cool.

Put the chopped cucumber into a strainer and sprinkle with salt. Let sit for 20 minutes to drain excess water.

Drop the spinach into a pot of boiling water, cook for 1 minute until bright green and wilted. Run under cold water and squeeze out excess water. Chop and set aside.

Chop the garlic with a generous pinch of salt, until it becomes a paste. Add the toasted cumin seeds and continue to chop. Transfer to a bowl and stir in the yogurt and 1 cup of water, until smooth. Stir in the wheat berries, cucumber, lemon juice, and mint.

Let chill for at least 2 hours and stir in the spinach right before eating.

Green Split Pea Soup

Ingredients

2 tablespoons olive oil

2 medium onions, chopped

2 dried bay leaves

1 cup carrots, diced

2 cups green split peas, picked through and rinsed

6 cups water, or stock

Salt, to taste

Half a lemon, juiced (optional)

Pepper, freshly ground

Preparation

Heat olive oil in a medium stockpot over medium-high heat. Add onions and cook until they soften. Add the bay leaves, carrot, split peas, and water. Bring to a boil, then reduce to a simmer. Simmer for 25 minutes, or until the split peas have softened but still have a bite. Season with salt to taste. Add more water if the soup is too thick.

Puree the soup, reserving about ¼ of the soup for a chunkier consistency. Heat through, taste for salt.

Stir in lemon juice, if using, and a few grinds of black pepper. Serve.

Chicken With Ginger Broth

Ingredients

4 chicken breasts, skinless, bone-in

1 (2-inch) piece fresh ginger, peeled and thinly sliced

3 leeks, white parts only

3 garlic cloves

Salt, to taste

2 cups daikon radishes or turnips, cut into large cubes (optional)

3 dried shiitake mushrooms, soaked in hot water

2 cups spinach, washed

1 tablespoon fresh cilantro

2 scallions, thinly sliced

Preparation

Put the chicken in a heavy pot with the ginger, daikon, and leeks. Add enough water to almost cover the chicken and sprinkle with salt. Bring to a boil, then cover and bring the heat to low. Simmer for 15 minutes, then turn the heat off and leave the chicken in the pot to steam for 30 minutes. Do not remove the lid.

While the chicken is steaming, drain the mushrooms, cut off the hard stalks, and thinly slice. Heat ½ cup water in a small saucepan and simmer the mushrooms for 5 minutes. Drain. Set aside.

Take the chicken from the pot and thinly slice the breasts. Bring the broth to a boil. Taste for salt.

Divide the spinach between 4 bowls. Add the mushrooms and then some sliced chicken. Cover with hot broth. Add a pinch of cilantro and scallions. Serve immediately.

Egg Noodles in Broth

Ingredients

6 cups homemade Chicken Stock or Basic Vegetable Stock

16 oz of egg nest pasta

4 cups of baby spinach

Parmesan cheese (optional)

Preparation

Bring the broth to a boil. Break the pasta into the broth and cook until just tender. Break up the pasta with a kitchen knife if you want the noodles shorter.

Stir in the spinach, and cook for 2 more minutes. Serve with a little Parmesan cheese, if desired.

Tarragon & Lemon Chicken Soup With Orzo

Ingredients

2 teaspoons olive oil

1 medium onion, chopped

2 stalks celery, cut into ¼-inch dice

2 medium carrots, cut into ¼-inch dice

Salt and pepper, to taste

6 cups of water

2 sprigs of tarragon

2 inch lemon peel

20 ounces chicken on the bone

½ cup orzo

1 tablespoon lemon juice

2 teaspoons tarragon leaves, chopped, for garnish

Preparation

In a heavy bottomed pot with a lid, heat the olive oil over medium heat. Add the onions, celery, carrots, and a sprinkle of salt. Cook for 5 to 8 minutes, or until the onions are translucent, do not let brown.

Add the 6 cups of water, tarragon sprigs, lemon peel, and chicken on the bone. Bring to a boil, then simmer for at least 40 minutes, skimming any foam or fat on the surfaces. Add a little water if the soup has reduced by more than 1 inch.

Remove the chicken and place into a bowl, let cool slightly then shred the meat and discard the bones. Return the chicken meat to the soup, bring to boil, then add in the orzo. Boil for 7 minutes then stir in the lemon juice, taste for seasonings then turn off the heat.

Ladle into bowls and serve with a sprinkling of fresh tarragon.

Matzo Ball Soup

Ingredients

For the matzo ball dough:

2 large eggs

1 tablespoons canola or grape seed oil

½ teaspoon salt

2 tablespoons cups seltzer

½ cup matzo meal (see Chef Tips)

For the soup:

1 tablespoon canola or grape seed oil

1 onion, finely chopped

1 stalk celery, chopped

2 parsnips, peeled and chopped

2 carrots, peeled and chopped

8 cups low-sodium chicken broth or Rich Chicken Stock

2 cups baby spinach, loosely packed

2 tablespoons fresh dill or flat leaf parsley, chopped

Preparation

Whisk the eggs in a medium bowl for 30 seconds or until foamy. Stir in oil, salt, and seltzer with a wooden spoon. Pour in the matzo meal in a steady stream while stirring. Gently fold in the matzo meal just moistened. Cover and chill in the refrigerator for at least 1 hour.

Meanwhile, in a large stockpot, heat oil and onions over medium-high heat. Once the onions have become translucent, add the celery. Cook, stirring occasionally, for 5 minutes. Add the carrots, parsnips, and chicken broth. Bring to a boil, then reduce to a simmer and cover.

Once the matzo dough has chilled, bring a pot of salted water to a boil. Reduce heat to a simmer. Using wet hands, very gently roll dough into loose balls, about 1 tablespoon in size. Drop them into the simmering water, one ball at a time. (Do not press the dough together tightly, as this will create heavier, denser matzo balls.) Cover and simmer for 30 minutes.

Once the matzo balls are ready, transfer to the chicken soup. Ladle into bowls, and serve with dill or parsley.

Gingery Carrot & Lentil Soup

Ingredients

3 large carrots, washed and scrubbed

1 medium onion, peeled and cut in half

2 tablespoons grapeseed or canola oil

1½ inch piece of fresh ginger root, peeled, and thinly sliced into matchsticks

1 clove of garlic, smashed, skin removed, and sliced

1 cup red lentils, picked through and rinsed

4 cups low-sodium vegetable or chicken stock

1 tablespoon lemon juice

Salt and pepper, to taste

Preparation

Top and tail the carrots. Cut them into pieces about 1½-inches long, then cut those pieces into 4 to 6 sticks, all about the same thickness for even cooking. Cut the onion halves into ⅓-inch slices lengthways. Set both aside.

Heat the oil in a heavy casserole or pan over a medium-high heat. Add the ginger and let it sizzle for a few moments, then add the garlic. Stir-fry until the garlic turns a very pale gold, infusing the oil.

Add the onions and saute until they begin to soften. Add the carrot sticks and saute for about 5 minutes, then turn the heat down to medium and partially cover the pan. Sweat the vegetables, stirring from time to time, until they are soft and have taken a golden color. This will take about 10 to 12 minutes. Do not let them burn!

Add the cleaned and rinsed lentils to the vegetables and mix them in well. Cook, stirring constantly for 1 minute. Add the stock, and turn the heat up to bring the soup to a boil. Cover, turn the heat down to low and simmer the soup until the lentils are soft and are easily mashed when pressed with the back of a spoon against the side of the pan, about 20 to 25 minutes. Blend the soup and return it to the pan. If the soup seems too thick, add a little more stock, water, or milk (unsweetened soy milk works well here too).

Add the lemon juice, mix, adjust for salt then heat gently until the soup starts to simmer. Turn the heat off, cover, and let the soup sit for 5 to 10 minutes. Serve with a liberal grinding of fresh black pepper on top and a swirl of yogurt if desired.

Hoppin' John

Ingredients

7 ½ cups of water, or vegetable stock, divided

1 cup brown basmati rice

1 bunch of spinach, or chard leaves, washed

2 tablespoons extra virgin olive oil

1 large onion, diced

3 dried sage leaves

Sea salt and black pepper, to taste

1 to 2 small, whole, dried chipotle chilies, or to taste

1 cup dried black eyed-peas, soaked over night in 3 times their volume of water, drained and rinsed

3 to 4 whole cloves of garlic, smashed and skinned

Preparation

In a small pot, bring the basmati rice and 1½ cups of stock or water to a boil. Simmer for 20 minutes, remove from heat, and set aside. (See Chef Tip)

Strip the leaves from the chard, roughly chop and set aside. Dice the stems.

In a Dutch oven, heat olive oil over medium-high heat. Add the onions, diced chard stems and sage leaves. Sautee for 2 minutes. Turn the heat down to medium, sprinkle with salt, and sautee the veggies for 5 to 8 minutes, partially covered.

Add the peas, chipotle and the garlic. Stir to mix and add enough water to cover. Bring to a boil. Reduce to a simmer and cook for 20 minutes. Add the partially cooked rice. Cook another 25 to 30 minutes until the beans are soft and the rice is al dente.

Add the chopped chard, stirring it in until it has completely wilted. Cover, turn off the heat and let the Hoppin" John stand for 5 to 10 minutes. Taste for salt, remove garlic, then serve with a grind or two of black pepper.

Cabbage Miso Soup

Ingredients

6 cups Basic Vegetable Stock or water

4 cups chopped green cabbage

2 celery ribs, sliced on a bias

1 yellow onion, halved and thinly sliced

1 carrot, thinly sliced (see Ann's Tips)

8 garlic cloves, 4 finely chopped and 4 sliced

⅓ cup red miso

Sesame oil (optional)

Preparation

Bring 6 cups of water or vegetable broth to a boil in a large soup pot. Add cabbage, celery, onion, carrot, and sliced garlic. Cover, reduce to medium-low heat, and cook for about 15 to 20 minutes, or until vegetables are tender.

Stir in chopped garlic, then turn off heat. Dissolve miso with some of the hot soup liquid in a cup or bowl, then pour it back into the pot. Ladle soup into bowls. For an extra zing of flavor, add a few drops of sesame oil to each bowl just before serving.

Fall Vegetable Soup With Spicy Gremolata

Ingredients

1 whole dried chipotle pepper pod, or ½ teaspoon of dried chipotle

1-pound kabocha or butter cup squash, seeded, and diced

½-pound onions or leeks, finely sliced

2 carrots, scrubbed and diced

6 garlic cloves, crushed and peeled

1-pound Yukon Gold potatoes, scrubbed, quartered lengthwise, and sliced to form a dice

½-pound green beans, topped, tailed, cut into ¾-inch lengths

½-pound zucchini, quartered lengthwise and thickly sliced to form a dice (optional)

1 bouquet garni (see Chef Tips)

2 teaspoons sea salt

2 (14-ounce) cans of cannellini beans, drained and rinsed

1 cup small whole wheat elbow macaroni

Freshly grated Parmesan, to taste (optional)

Pepper, to taste

1 recipe Spicy Gremolata

Preparation

Place all of the soup vegetables into a large pot, except for the canned beans and the macaroni.

Add the bouquet garni and 3 quarts of water, or enough to cover the vegetables by 1-inch. Add the salt. Bring to a boil, cover and let simmer gently for an hour or until the vegetables are tender and the squash can be mashed against the sides of the pan. While the soup is cooking, prepare the Spicy Gremolata (to learn how, click here).

Remove the bouquet garni. Mash some of the squash against the pan to thicken the broth. Add the beans, cook for 10 minutes. Taste for salt. Add the macaroni. Cook until al dente. Stir in the Spicy Herb Pesto and serve immediately with the grated cheese.

Clear Pumpkin Soup

Ingredients

3 teaspoons instant dashi powder (see Chef Tips)

1 cup sake or dry sherry

2 tablespoons mirin

1 cup soy sauce (see Chef Tips)

2 tablespoons sugar

6 cups water

2 tablespoons ginger, minced

2 cups potatoes, peeled and diced

1 small cheese pumpkin or kabocha, about 3 cups, peeled and diced

1 carrot, peeled and diced

1 onion, diced

½ cup scallions, chopped

Preparation

Bring the dashi, sherry, mirin, soy, sugar, water, and ginger to a simmer.

Add the potatoes, pumpkin, carrots, and onions to the pot, simmer until the vegetables are soft, about 30 minutes.

Garnish with chopped scallions

Curried Coconut Carrot Soup

Ingredients

1 tablespoon canola, or grape seed oil

1 medium onion, chopped

2 teaspoons red curry paste

2 tablespoons fresh ginger, peeled and chopped

2 garlic cloves, minced

2 pounds carrots, peeled and cut in into ½-inch pieces

Salt, to taste

3 cups water, or stock

1 (14 ounce) can coconut milk

Cilantro, for garnish

Preparation

In a medium stockpot, heat the oil over medium-high heat. Add the onion and cook for 5 minutes or until translucent. Add the curry paste, ginger, and garlic. Stir for 2 minutes.

Add the carrots and a generous pinch of salt. Cover and let the carrots steam for 5 minutes, stirring occasionally. Uncover and add the water or broth and coconut milk. Bring to a boil. Cover and simmer for at least 30 minutes, or until the carrots are soft.

Puree soup, until very smooth. Heat through, adding more water if the soup is too thick. Serve with a cilantro stem.

Wonton Soup With Shiitake Mushrooms

Ingredients

2 quarts low-sodium vegetable stock

¼ cup low-sodium soy sauce

1 (¼ inch) slice ginger

1 garlic clove

1 cup shiitake mushrooms, sliced

1 bunch scallions, sliced, white and green sections divided

8 chicken dumplings, prepared

Preparation

In a medium sauce pot, bring the vegetable stock, soy sauce, ginger and garlic to a boil. Reduce the heat to a simmer and cook for 15 minutes.

Add the mushrooms and white part of the scallions to the soup. Cook for another 10 minutes or until the mushrooms are soft.

Add the frozen dumplings and cook for about 4 or 5 minutes until they are cooked through. Remove the garlic and ginger from the soup and serve. Garnish with the rest of the scallions.

Summer Borscht

Ingredients

2 pounds beets, washed and scrubbed

1 cup grated cucumber

3 scallion stalks, white and light green parts only, chopped

3 tablespoons chopped dill

2 cups plain yogurt

1 tablespoon sugar

1 large lemon, juiced

1 tablespoon white or red wine vinegar

Salt and pepper, to taste

Preparation

Bring 6 cups of water and the beets to a boil. Simmer until the beets are tender, about 20 to 30 minutes, depending on size. Remove the beets and strain the cooking liquid into a measuring cup. Let the beets and the cooking liquid cool.

Once the beets are cooled, peel and grate them. In a large bowl mix the grated beets with the shredded cucumber, chopped scallions, dill, yogurt, lemon juice, vinegar and salt and pepper. Pour in 1 cup of the beet cooking liquid, mix well, adding more liquid for a looser soup. Keep in the refrigerator for at least 30 minutes before serving.

Pumpkin Miso Soup

Ingredients

1 small kabocha pumpkin, washed, halved, and seeds scraped out

2 tablespoon grapeseed or canola oil

1 large Spanish onion, thinly sliced

8 to 10 cups low-sodium stock or water

2 to 3 tablespoons yellow miso paste (miso shiro), or to taste

Sea salt and black pepper, to taste

Soy sauce (optional)

Preparation

With a peeler, take off little patches of skin all over the pumpkin halves until they look polka dotted. This is purely decorative and can be left out if you don't have time. Cut the halves into a ½-inch dice. Set aside.

Heat the oil in a large soup pot over a medium-high heat. When it ripples, add the onion and saute, stirring until the onion starts to soften and turn transparent. Add the pumpkin cubes, sprinkle with a little sea salt, mix well, and cover. Turn the heat down to medium low and sweat the vegetables for about 10 minutes, or until the pumpkin has started to soften and the onion is soft. The onion should not brown, so stir the pot occasionally to make sure it doesn't stick.

Add enough stock to the pot to cover the vegetables plus 1 inch. Raise the heat and bring to a boil. Cover, turn the heat to low, and simmer until the pumpkin is soft but not mushy, about 10 minutes. Do not overcook! While the soup is cooking, measure the miso into a bowl. Using a small balloon whisk or a fork, gradually whisk in ½ cup of warm stock or cool water until you have a thinnish, creamy-looking liquid with no lumps.

When the pumpkin is tender, add a grind or two of black pepper and turn off the heat. Add the miso cream little by little, stirring gently to mix. Taste as you go until you know how much you like. Miso is richly salty, so you do not want too much in the soup. Check for seasoning. Serve immediately.

Roasted Garlic Soup

Ingredients

18 garlic cloves, in skin

1 tablespoon olive oil

1 cup chopped onion

10 fresh garlic cloves, smashed and chopped

Salt and pepper, to taste

1 heaping teaspoon freshly chopped sage

1 heaping teaspoon fresh thyme

3½ cups of water or broth

½ cup grated parmesan

½ cup freshly grated Parmesan cheese, plus more for serving

4 chunks of good stale bread

Fresh grind of black pepper

Preparation

Preheat the oven to 350 degrees. Place the garlic in a ceramic baking pan, drizzle with olive oil, and sprinkle with salt. Cover with foil and bake in the oven for 40 minutes until soft. Squeeze out the garlic into a bowl.

In a heavy bottomed pot, heat the 1 tablespoon of olive oil. Add the onions and cook over medium-low heat for 5 to 8 minutes or until translucent. Add in the roasted garlic, fresh garlic, sage, thyme and a generous pinch of salt. Cook for another 3 minutes.

Add in the water or broth and the piece of Parmesan rind. Bring to a boil, and then simmer for at least 20 minutes. Puree with an immersion blender. Stir in the freshly grated Parmesan cheese, then taste for seasonings.

Before serving, place the chunks of bread in the bottom of four bowls. Ladle the soup over the bread, then grind fresh pepper. Serve immediately with some extra grated cheese.

Quick Posole

Ingredients

2 teaspoons dried oregano, divided

1 red onion, chopped, divided

3½ cups low-sodium chicken broth, divided

⅛ teaspoon salt

1 clove garlic, finely chopped

1 teaspoon ground red chile, or chili powder

1 (15-ounce) can yellow or white hominy, rinsed

1 (15-ounce) can black beans, rinsed

12 ounces boneless, skinless chicken breasts, trimmed and cut into ¾-inch pieces

1 cup shredded green cabbage, for garnish (see Chef Tips)

1 lime, cut into wedges, for garnish

Preparation

In a small skillet over medium-high heat, toast oregano until fragrant, about 30 to 40 seconds. Transfer to a saucepan to cool.

Combine one teaspoon oregano with ¼ cup onion and set aside.

Combine the remaining onion with ¼ cup broth and salt. Cover and cook over medium heat until the onion is translucent. Add garlic and cook for one minute. Add the remaining teaspoon of oregano and ground chile or chili powder and cook for an additional minute.

Add the hominy and remaining broth. Bring to a simmer and cook for five minutes. Add the black beans and chicken, return to a simmer and cook until the chicken is no longer pink in the center, about five minutes.

Serve in bowls, garnished with cabbage, the reserved onion-oregano mixture, and a squeeze of lime.

Turmeric Dal

Ingredients

2 cups split red lentils picked over and washed well

4 cups water

½ inch ginger root peeled and quartered

½ teaspoon of turmeric

salt to taste

For the spiced oil:

2 tablespoons ghee, butter (see Chef Tips), or coconut oil

2 teaspoons cumin seeds

2 cloves garlic, sliced through the root

1 to 2 whole dried red chilies (or to taste)

2 tablespoons cilantro, chopped (optional)

Preparation

Put the lentils, water, ginger, and turmeric into a heavy pot with a lid. Bring to a boil, skimming off any scum that forms on top. Add salt to taste. Turn the heat down to low and cover.

Simmer until the lentils are soft and breaking up, about 25 to 30 minutes. Keep an eye on them as they thicken and soften, they will need stirring to stop them sticking to the bottom of the pan. When they are thick and creamy looking, remove from the heat, and discard the ginger. Cover and set aside.

Heat the ghee in a small skillet over medium-high heat. When it has completely melted, and starts to ripple, add the cumin seeds. Cook for 30 seconds. Add the garlic and chili pods. Cook stirring until the garlic colors and the chili pods have darkened to a deep red. Add the cilantro. It will spit and sizzle. Cook for a few seconds then tip the spiced oil over the lentils. Mix well and serve immediately with Brown Basmati Rice.

Broccoli & Almond Soup

Ingredients

½ cup whole blanched almonds

1 tablespoon olive oil

½ of a medium leek, white and green parts only, halved lengthwise and sliced

½ pound Yukon Gold potato (about 2 medium), peeled and cubed

1 tablespoon chopped fresh thyme, plus more for garnish

1 clove garlic, minced

4 cups stock or water

4 loose cups broccoli florets (about ½ a medium head), stems included – peeled and cubed

Salt and fresh ground pepper, to taste

½ cup freshly grated Parmesan, plus more garnish

Preparation

Toast the almonds in a skillet until they make popping noises or their skin has darkened and fragrant. Remove from heat immediately and pour into a bowl. Set aside.

Heat olive oil in a saucepan over medium heat. Add leeks, potatoes and thyme. Cook until the leeks have softened. Add garlic and cook for 3 minutes.

Add stock or water and bring to a boil. Turn the heat back down to medium. Simmer until the potatoes are tender. Remove 1 cup of stock and puree with almonds. Set aside.

Add broccoli and salt and cook for 3 minutes or until the broccoli is bright green. In batches in a blender, or with a hand blender, puree the soup. Return to the saucepan, and stir in the almond puree, Parmesan, and black pepper. Heat through.

Serve with fresh thyme, black pepper, and some Parmesan cheese.

Cold Roasted Red Pepper Soup

Ingredients

1 pound vine-ripened tomatoes, quartered

2 large red peppers, seeded and cut into 2 inch slices

2 tablespoons olive oil, divided

Salt and pepper, to taste

1 yellow onion, chopped

2 cloves of garlic, minced

½ teaspoon ground coriander

Juice from ½ a lemon

Chopped fresh mint

Preparation

Preheat the oven to 350 degrees.

In a large bowl, toss the tomatoes and red peppers with 1 tablespoon of olive oil, salt, and pepper until coated with oil. Transfer to a baking sheet. Cook until the vegetables are browned in spots and tender, about 30 minutes.

Meanwhile, in a sauté pan, heat the remaining 1 tablespoon of olive oil. Add the onions and garlic, and cook until the onions have turned translucent, about 7-10 minutes. Add the coriander, and cook stirring for 1 minute. Turn off the heat and let sit until the roasted tomatoes and peppers are done.

Puree the onion mixture with the roasted tomatoes and pepper, along with ½ to 1 cup of water. Puree until smooth.

Let the soup sit at room temperature uncovered for about 30 minutes then chill in the refrigerator for at least 2 hours. Stir in lemon juice and chopped mint and serve cold.

Spanish Garlic Soup

Ingredients

2 tablespoons olive oil

¼ pound any stale bread, crusts removed, cut into 1/2 inch cubes (see Chef Tips)

4 garlic cloves, minced

½ teaspoon hot pimentón (smoked paprika)

Salt, to taste

4 cups chicken stock or vegetable stock

4 eggs, poached

Preparation

In a medium-sized pot, heat the olive oil over medium-high heat. Add the cubed bread and cook for 5 minutes, stirring often, until the bread is lightly browned. Add the garlic, pimentón, and a pinch of salt. Stir well, and cook for 3 minutes.

Pour in the stock, bring to a boil, then reduce heat to a simmer. Cook for 15 minutes, or longer for a sweeter less pungent garlic flavor.

Ladle soup into bowls and serve topped with a freshly poached egg.

Fish Sticks With Lemon Mayo

Ingredients

Fish Sticks

1¼ pound white fish fillets such as cod, snapper, bass, halibut or hake

Juice from ½ a lemon

1 cup panko breadcrumbs

¼ cup cornmeal

1 teaspoon salt

Ground black pepper, to taste

2 tablespoons olive oil

2 eggs

Lemon Mayonnaise:

⅓ cup mayonnaise

2-3 teaspoons freshly squeezed lemon juice, or to taste

¼ teaspoon hot paprika (optional)

Preparation

Preheat the oven to 425 degrees. Line a baking tray with parchment paper. Set aside.

Cut the fish fillets into 1-inch strips lengthwise, and then in half horizontally. Let sit in a bowl with lemon juice for 5 minutes.

Meanwhile, in a medium bowl mix together the panko, cornmeal, salt, pepper and olive oil. Mix well.

In a separate bowl, lightly beat the eggs. Pat the fish dry and dip into the eggs, allowing the excess to drip off. Then dip into the panko mixture, pressing to cover the fish evenly with the breadcrumbs. Repeat and transfer to the prepared baking sheet, allowing space between the breaded fish.

Bake until the fish is cooked through and the crust is golden, about 20-25 minutes, turning halfway through.

While the fish is baking, put the mayonnaise into a small bowl. Beat in the lemon juice one teaspoon at a time, until desired consistency and flavor. Beat in the paprika, if using.

If not serving the fish sticks right away, transfer to a wire rack. Serve with the lemon mayo.

Easy White Rice

Ingredients

2 cups long-grain white rice

3 cups water

Salt, to taste

Preparation

Place the rice, water, and salt in a heavy pot with a tight-fitting lid. Bring to a rolling boil. Cover the pot and turn the heat down to low. Simmer the rice gently for 20 minutes. Do not lift the lid.

Turn the heat off. Keep the rice covered and leave the rice to steam for 10 to 15 minutes. No peeking! Fluff with a fork and serve.

Vegan Hot Chocolate

Ingredients

4 cups soy, almond, or oat milk (plain, unsweetened)

2 tablespoons chocolate protein powder

3 tablespoons cocoa powder

2 tablespoons agave nectar, or to taste

Preparation

In a small sauce pot, heat almond milk on medium low heat. Add protein powder and cocoa powder and whisk until powders are combined with the milk.

Add the agave and stir. Heat until warm and serve.

Spicy Turkey Posole

Ingredients

1 dried chipotle pepper

½ teaspoon ground cumin

1 teaspoon chili powder

6 garlic cloves

2 cups chopped onions, divided

2 tablespoons olive oil

1 pound turkey thighs

1 teaspoon dried oregano

1 (14.5-ounce) can hominy, drained and rinsed

½ cup fresh cilantro, chopped

1 cup red cabbage, thinly sliced

½ radish, thinly sliced

Salt and pepper, to taste

Baked tortilla strips

6 (8½-inch) whole wheat or corn tortillas

Olive oil, as needed

Salt to taste

Preparation

In a small pot, bring 2 cups of water to a boil. Remove from heat, add chile pepper and let steep until plump.

In a blender, process the chili peppers, ground cumin, chili powder, garlic cloves, 1 cup onion, and 1 cup water until smooth. Strain through a sieve and reserve liquid.

In a large pot over medium heat, heat olive oil. Add remaining onions and sauté for about 5 minutes, or until translucent. Season with salt and pepper.

Add turkey thighs and oregano. Cover with 10 cups water and chili liquid. Bring to a boil then reduce to a simmer. Simmer the soup for about 30 minutes, or until turkey is thoroughly cooked and fork-tender.

Remove turkey from pot and shred with two forks. Return turkey to pot and add hominy. Cook for another 5 minutes until turkey and hominy are warmed through.

For the baked tortilla strips: Preheat the oven to 375 degrees. Brush both sides of the tortillas with oil, then stack and cut into strips of desired size. Arrange tortilla pieces on a baking sheet and bake until crispy and browned, about 8 to 10 minutes.

Serve in bowls and garnish with tortilla strips, cilantro, red cabbage, and radishes.

Banana Coconut Smoothie

Ingredients

¾ cup coconut milk

1 small frozen banana (see Chef Tips)

1 teaspoon honey

2 ice cubes

2 tablespoons water, as needed

Preparation

Combine all ingredients in a blender, and blend until smooth. Taste for sweetness then serve immediately.

Ginger Tea

Ingredients

1 inch chunk of ginger, peeled and cut into thin slices

2 cups of water

Lemon juice (optional)

Honey or brown sugar, to taste

Preparation

In a small stockpot, boil the ginger with water. Reduce to a simmer and steep for 5-10 minutes depending on desired strength.

Remove from heat and stir in lemon juice, if using, and honey or sugar to taste. Drink immediately or chill.

Italian Wedding Soup

Ingredients

¾ pound ground chicken

⅔ cup breadcrumbs

1 large egg

¾ cup parmesan cheese, freshly grated, divided

1 tablespoon fresh oregano, chopped

1 teaspoon lemon zest

1 garlic clove, minced

¼ teaspoon red pepper flakes (optional)

Salt and pepper, to taste

1 tablespoon olive oil

4 cups chicken stock

6 kale leaves, stems removed, roughly chopped

Preparation

In a bowl, mix together the ground chicken, breadcrumbs, egg, parmesan, oregano, lemon zest, garlic, red pepper flakes, salt and pepper. Form into 1-inch balls.

Heat 1 tablespoon of olive oil in a wide skillet over medium-high heat. Cook the meatballs until evenly golden brown, they do not need to be cooked all the way through as they will finish cooking in the soup. Transfer the meatballs to a plate covered with a plate lined with paper towels.

Heat the chicken stock and bring to a boil. Add the kale leaves and the meatballs. Simmer for 15 minutes. Stir in ¼ cup of parmesan cheese. Taste the broth for seasonings then serve.

Peach of a Carrot Zucchini Smoothie

Ingredients

1 medium peach, unpeeled, halved and pitted (fresh, frozen, or unsweetened canned)

1 small carrot, unpeeled and chopped into quarters

½ small zucchini or yellow summer squash, unpeeled and chopped into quarters

2 tablespoons pumpkin seeds, unsalted

½ teaspoon cinnamon

½ cup milk of choice

½ teaspoon vanilla extract

5 ice cubes

Preparation

Place peach, carrot, and squash in the container of a blender. Then add pumpkin seeds, cinnamon, milk, vanilla extract, and ice cubes.

Cover and process for a few seconds until smooth and creamy.

Pour into a glass and enjoy immediately, or chill until serving time.

Creamy Cashew & Pineapple Green Smoothie

Ingredients

½ cup cashews

1 cup pineapple chunks, frozen (see Chef Tips)

1 cup kale, de-stemmed and torn into pieces

½ medium apple, cut into chunks

1 ½ – 2 cups milk (dairy or plant-based)

Preparation

Place the cashews in a bowl or small container and add enough water to cover them by a half-inch. Transfer to the fridge to soak overnight (see Chef Tips).

Drain the water from the cashews. Add all ingredients, including 1 ½ cups of milk, to a high-speed blender and blend on high until smooth. Add another ½ cup of milk to thin the smoothie if needed.

Serve immediately.

Cocoa Cherry Protein Shake

Ingredients

¾ cup whole milk

¼ cup Greek yogurt

½ cup frozen cherries

1 tbsp protein powder (see Chef Notes)

1 tbsp unsweetened cocoa powder

1 tbsp nut butter

1 tbsp flaxseed meal

½ cup ice

Preparation

Add all ingredients to a high-speed blender and blend on high until smooth. Serve immediately.

Mixed Berry Smoothie

Ingredients

1 cup frozen blackberries

½ cup frozen raspberries

½ avocado

½ cup Greek yogurt

1 cup whole milk

1 tbsp honey

½ tsp vanilla extract

Preparation

Add all ingredients to a high-speed blender and blend on high until smooth.

Serve immediately.

Banana Oat Smoothie

Ingredients

1 cup whole milk

1 tbsp nut butter

1 large banana

5-6 ice cubes

¼ cup rolled oats

½ tsp vanilla extract

¼ cup protein powder (see Chef Notes)

½ tsp cinnamon

Pinch of nutmeg

1 tbsp flaxseed meal

1 tbsp honey

Preparation

Add all ingredients to a high-speed blender and blend on high until smooth.

Serve immediately.

Chocolate Avocado Smoothie

Ingredients

1 ½ cups whole milk

1 banana

½ avocado

1 cup spinach

2 tbsp cocoa powder

1 tbsp honey or maple syrup

1 tbsp hemp seeds

½ tsp cinnamon

A pinch of nutmeg

A pinch of salt

Preparation

Add all ingredients to a high-speed blender and blend on high until smooth.

Serve immediately.

Tropical Protein Smoothie

Ingredients

1 Navel orange

½ cup full fat coconut milk

¼ cup protein powder (see Chef Notes)

1 banana

½ avocado

½ cup ice

Preparation

Add all ingredients to a high-speed blender and blend on high until smooth.

Serve immediately.

High Protein Blueberry Smoothie

Ingredients

1 ½ cups blueberries

½ cup whole milk

½ cup spinach

½ banana

¼ cup protein powder (see Chef Notes)

½ cup Greek yogurt

½ rolled oats

Preparation

Add all ingredients to a high-speed blender and blend on high until smooth.

Serve immediately.

Tahini Shake

Ingredients

2 bananas, peeled, sliced, and frozen

1 cup whole milk

¼ tablespoons tahini

4 dates, pitted or 1 tablespoon maple syrup

1½ cups ice

1 teaspoon vanilla extract

1 teaspoon cinnamon (optional)

Preparation

Place all ingredients in a blender and blend on high until smooth. Pour into two glasses and garnish with sliced bananas and cinnamon.

Cold Beet Soup with Honeyed Ricotta

Ingredients

2 quarts vegetable stock

2 large beets, peeled and chopped

2 sprigs rosemary

4 sprigs thyme

1 cup ricotta cheese

½ cup Greek yogurt

2 tablespoons honey

1 cup balsamic vinegar

Salt and pepper to taste

Preparation

In a large pot over high heat, combine stock, beets, rosemary, and thyme. Bring to a boil and cook beets until very tender, about 25 minutes. Once beets are cooked, allow to cool. Blend soup until very smooth and season with salt and pepper. Refrigerate until chilled.

In a small bowl, mix together ricotta, yogurt, and honey. Season with salt and pepper. Set aside to chill.

In a small pot, bring balsamic vinegar to a simmer. Reduce by half. Set aside to cool.

When you are ready to eat, serve each bowl of beet soup with a dollop of ricotta mixture swirled in, and a drizzle of the reduced balsamic vinegar.

Lavender Lemonade

Ingredients

9 cups water, divided

1 cup sugar

¼ cup dried lavender blossoms

1 cup lemon juice

Preparation

In a small pot over medium high heat, combine sugar, lavender, and 1 cup water.

Strain lavender syrup into a large pitcher. Add lemon juice and 8 cups water. Adjust to taste, adding more lemon juice or water as necessary.

Chill and serve over ice.

Sweet Potato Hummus

Ingredients

1 lb sweet potato, peeled and cut into 1-inch chunks (1-2 sweet potatoes, depending on their size)

1 (15 ounce) can chickpeas, rinsed

½ cup sesame tahini

¾ cup of olive oil, divided

Salt and pepper

4 sprigs parsley, leaves roughly chopped (optional)

Preparation

Bring a pot of water to a boil. Add the sweet potato and cook until fork-tender, about 15 to 20 minutes. Reserve 1 cup of the cooking liquid. Drain. Let the potatoes cool slightly.

In a food processor, combine the cooked sweet potato, chickpeas, salt, pepper, and tahini. Purée until smooth. Slowly add 2/3 cup of the olive oil to the puree, pulsing all the while. If the mixture looks too stiff, add the reserved cooking liquid as needed.

Top with fresh chopped parsley and drizzle with the remaining olive oil. Serve with warm pita, or steamed or raw vegetables.

Roasted Cauliflower Steaks With Sunflower Seed Pesto

Ingredients

Cauliflower Steaks

1 large cauliflower, cut into 3-4 (1-inch-thick) whole slices, plus remaining florets (see Chef Tips)

3 teaspoons olive oil, divided

Salt and black pepper, to taste

1 teaspoon chopped fresh thyme, plus a few stems for garnish

Sunflower Seed Pesto

¼ cup olive oil

⅓ cup packed fresh basil leaves, plus more for garnish

¼ cup raw or dry roasted and unsalted shelled sunflower seeds, plus more for garnish

1 teaspoon Dijon mustard

1 teaspoon honey

½ clove garlic, peeled

Salt and ground black pepper, to taste

Preparation

Preheat oven to 425 degrees.

Line a large rimmed baking sheet with parchment paper or aluminum foil. (If using foil, spray with nonstick cooking spray.) Place cauliflower on prepared baking sheet, and brush "steaks" and florets with 2 teaspoons of oil. Sprinkle with pinch of salt and pepper. Roast until lightly caramelized and almost cooked through, about 18 minutes.

Gently flip each "steak" and floret and brush with 1 more teaspoon of oil. Sprinkle with thyme, a pinch of salt and pepper and roast until well caramelized and cooked through, about 10 more minutes.

While cauliflower is roasting, prepare the pesto. Place olive oil, basil, sunflower seeds, mustard, honey, and garlic in bowl of a small food processor and pulse until smooth. Season with salt and pepper to taste, and pulse a few more times until well combined and desired flavor is achieved.

Arrange cauliflower on large plate or platter. Top with pesto, and garnish with sunflower seeds, thyme, and basil.

Peach of a Carrot Zucchini Smoothie

Ingredients

1 medium peach, unpeeled, halved and pitted (fresh, frozen, or unsweetened canned)

1 small carrot, unpeeled and chopped into quarters

½ small zucchini or yellow summer squash, unpeeled and chopped into quarters

2 tablespoons pumpkin seeds, unsalted

½ teaspoon cinnamon

½ cup milk of choice

½ teaspoon vanilla extract

5 ice cubes

Preparation

Place peach, carrot, and squash in the container of a blender. Then add pumpkin seeds, cinnamon, milk, vanilla extract, and ice cubes.

Cover and process for a few seconds until smooth and creamy.

Pour into a glass and enjoy immediately, or chill until serving time.

Spinach Saag

Ingredients

2 tablespoons olive oil

1 onion, finely chopped

¼ cup ginger, minced

2 cloves garlic, minced

1 serrano pepper, minced, or to taste (see Chef Tips)

1 teaspoon garam masala

2 teaspoons ground coriander

1 teaspoon ground cumin

1 pound fresh baby spinach

¼ cup plain yogurt

Preparation

Heat the oil in a saute pan over medium heat. Add the onions, ginger, garlic, and serrano and saute for 5 minutes until the mixture is aromatic. Add the garam masala, coriander, and cumin, then cook for another 5 minutes until onions are translucent but not burnt.

Add the spinach and stir well, incorporating the spiced onion mixture into the spinach. Add salt and pepper to taste. Cook until the spinach is wilted.

Turn the heat off. Stir in the yogurt into the spinach until well mixed.

Miso Polenta

Ingredients

4¼ cups water

1 cup polenta

1 tablespoon miso paste, plus

2 teaspoons miso paste

1/8 teaspoon garlic powder

1/8 teaspoon ground ginger

2 green onions, chopped, to garnish (optional)

Sesame seeds, to garnish (optional)

Preparation

In a medium saucepan, bring water to a boil.

Add polenta gradually and whisk until there are no lumps. Lower the heat to low and cook, uncovered, until the mixture thickens, about 20 to 25 minutes. It is important to stir the polenta every five minutes or so to ensure that the bottom of the pan does not burn.

Turn off the heat and add the miso, garlic powder, and ground ginger. Whisk to combine. Serve immediately and garnish with green onions and sesame seeds, if using.

Tropical Protein Smoothie

Ingredients

1 Navel orange

½ cup full fat coconut milk

¼ cup protein powder (see Chef Notes)

1 banana

½ avocado

½ cup ice

Preparation

Add all ingredients to a high-speed blender and blend on high until smooth.

Serve immediately.

Vegan Pho

Ingredients

For broth:

1 quart vegetable stock store bought or homemade

3 tablespoons fresh ginger, sliced

1 teaspoon miso

1 tablespoon soy sauce

1 jalapeno pepper, thinly sliced

For soup:

1 6 oz. package rice stick noodles (see Chef Tips)

1 half carrot, very thinly sliced

1 leek, julienned

¼ cup sweet corn, off the cob

2 shitake mushrooms, very thinly sliced

Cilantro leaves, for garnish

Preparation

In a medium saucepan, heat stock to a simmer. Stir in the miso and soy. Steep the ginger and a few slices of the jalapeno in the broth for 5 minutes and then strain if desired. If you like spicy food, simply leave them in.

Separately, in a medium-sized pot, boil rice noodles until still al dente. Transfer noodles to bowls.

Garnish noodles with chopped vegetables and cilantro leaves.

Bring broth to a boil and pour directly over the noodles. The boiling broth will lightly cook the vegetables.

Apple Pie Smoothie

Ingredients

½ cup applesauce

¾ cup very cold plain Greek yogurt

¼ teaspoon freshly grated nutmeg

¼ teaspoon cinnamon

¼ teaspoon ground ginger (see Chef Tips)

Pinch allspice

1 teaspoon maple syrup, or to taste

3 tablespoons apple juice or water, as needed

Preparation

Combine all ingredients in a blender and blend until smooth, adding an ice cube or two if your ingredients are not very cold. Taste for sweetness and consistency, then drink immediately.

Chicken & Rice Congee

Ingredients

2 half skinless chicken breasts on the bone (see Chef Tips)

4 skinless chicken thighs on the bone

10 cups chicken stock or water

3 (¼-inch thick) slices fresh ginger

3 scallions, halved crosswise and smashed with flat side of a heavy knife

½ teaspoon salt

1 cup long-grain white or brown rice

Preparation

Bring chicken and broth (or water) to a boil in a large 10-cup pot. Add ginger and scallions and simmer, uncovered, for 20 minutes or until breast meat is cooked, skimming off foam occasionally. Transfer the two chicken halves with tongs to a bowl. Continue cooking the thighs in the broth for another 40 minutes.

When the breast meat has cooled completely remove the bones and tear the meat into shreds. Keep covered in the fridge until ready to use. Bring to room temperature before serving.

Strain the stock through a large sieve into a large bowl. Discard solids and wipe the cooking pot clean. You should have about 8 cups: if less, add water; if more, cook longer after adding rice. Return stock to the cleaned pot and check for salt. Add the rice.

Bring to a boil and stir. Reduce heat to low. Simmer covered stirring from time to time, until the rice is the consistency of oatmeal, about 1½-1¾ hours. If you have a heat diffuser, slip it under the pot to slow the cooking. Stir frequently during last ½ hour of cooking as the congee will be thick and tend to stick. Congee will continue to thicken as it stands, so thin with water if necessary.

Season congee with salt to taste. Serve topped with chicken and accompaniments to taste, such as chopped scallions, soy sauce, poached or hard boiled egg, salted roast peanuts or pickled vegetables.

Bananas En Papillote

Ingredients

2 bananas, halved lengthwise then halved across

1/2 lemon, juiced

2 teaspoons butter

2 teaspoons honey

2 teaspoons chopped pistachios

1/2 teaspoon fresh gingerroot, peeled and thinly sliced

2 large pieces of parchment paper

Preparation

Preheat oven to 400F.

Place half of all ingredients on top of one piece of parchment and repeat process with the second piece of parchment paper.

Wrap up your first parchment by folding the left and right corners of the paper toward the center, creasing the edges shut as tightly as you can. Next, fold and crease the top and bottom edges toward the center. Repeat for the second package.

Bake on a sheet pan for 5 minutes until well heated through and very aromatic. Cut the paper open right before eating and serve immediately.

Peanut Butter & Banana Smoothie

Ingredients

½ cup fat-free milk

½ cup plain non-fat Greek yogurt

1 tablespoon peanut butter

2 cups fresh spinach

1 medium banana

Directions

Combine ingredients in a blender and blend until smooth.

Poultry Bone Stock

Ingredients

1 chicken or turkey carcass

1 medium onion, peeled

3 garlic cloves

1 large carrot, scrubbed, topped, and tailed

1 rib of celery, cut in half

4 sprigs of parsley

1 bay leaf

1 teaspoon whole black peppercorns

1 teaspoon sea salt, or to taste

Preparation

Put the carcass into a large pot and cover with cold water.

Stick the cloves into the onion. Cut the carrots in half, and then into quarters lengthwise.

Put the onions, carrots, and celery in the pot with the chicken bones. Add the bay leaves, peppercorns, and 6 quarts of cold water. Bring to a boil and add 1 teaspoon sea salt, partially cover, and reduce the heat to low. Simmer for 1½ - 2 hours or until the bones have fallen apart. If you have a pressure cooker, an hour of cooking in the pressure cooker is equal to 3-4 hours simmering on the stove.

Strain the stock through a fine sieve into a clean pot and bring to a boil and reduce by about one quarter. Taste stock for salt, strain again into a container and chill in the fridge.

Remove any yellow fat that has formed on the top of the stock. Store in the fridge and use within 3 days or store in the freezer. Try using the stock in our Leftover Turkey Minestrone Soup.

Banana Pudding

 Ingredients

2 ripe bananas (see Chef Tips)

1 tablespoons cane sugar

1 tablespoons corn starch

Pinch sea salt

1 1/4 cup milk

2 egg yolks

¼ teaspoon vanilla extract

Shortbread cookies (optional)

Preparation

Preheat the oven to 350 degrees. Bake 1 banana in its skin on a baking sheet for about 30 minutes, or until the skin has burst. Carefully peel and mash. Set aside. Peel and slice the other banana, set aside.

Off the heat, in a small saucepan, mix the sugar, cornstarch, and salt. Gradually whisk in the milk, making sure the cornstarch does not clump. Whisk in the egg yolks.

Turn the heat onto medium, and heat the custard. Stir constantly until the custard begins to thicken and bubble, about 10-15 minutes. Be patient — don't turn up the heat, just keep stirring and it will suddenly thicken. Turn the heat down to low and cook for 1 more minute.

Remove the custard from the heat and stir in the mashed banana and vanilla extract. Pour the entire mixture into a shallow bowl then top with reserved sliced bananas or if using cookies, pour just enough to cover the bottom. Layer with banana slices and wafers, then cover with custard. Repeat the layers, ending with the custard on top.

Chill for at least 1 hour. Serve.

Chicken With Ginger Broth

Ingredients

4 chicken breasts, skinless, bone-in

1 (2-inch) piece fresh ginger, peeled and thinly sliced

3 leeks, white parts only

3 garlic cloves

Salt, to taste

2 cups daikon radishes or turnips, cut into large cubes (optional)

3 dried shiitake mushrooms, soaked in hot water

2 cups spinach, washed

1 tablespoon fresh cilantro

2 scallions, thinly sliced

Preparation

Put the chicken in a heavy pot with the ginger, daikon, and leeks. Add enough water to almost cover the chicken and sprinkle with salt. Bring to a boil, then cover and bring the heat to low. Simmer for 15 minutes, then turn the heat off and leave the chicken in the pot to steam for 30 minutes. Do not remove the lid.

While the chicken is steaming, drain the mushrooms, cut off the hard stalks, and thinly slice. Heat ½ cup water in a small saucepan and simmer the mushrooms for 5 minutes. Drain. Set aside.

Take the chicken from the pot and thinly slice the breasts. Bring the broth to a boil. Taste for salt.

Divide the spinach between 4 bowls. Add the mushrooms and then some sliced chicken. Cover with hot broth. Add a pinch of cilantro and scallions. Serve immediately.

Chicken & Noodles in Coconut Lime Broth

Ingredients

2 teaspoons canola oil

½ onion, sliced thin

1 clove garlic, sliced thin

3-inch piece ginger, peeled and cut into slices

¼ teaspoon red pepper flakes, or to taste

4 cups chicken broth

2 cups coconut milk

2 teaspoons lime zest

2 teaspoons fish sauce

½ pound shiitake mushrooms, sliced (about 2 cups)

6 ounces flat rice noodles

10 ounces skinless, boneless chicken breast, sliced into thin strips

½ cup loosely packed baby spinach or roughly chopped spinach

¼ cup fresh lime juice

2 tablespoons cilantro leaves, roughly chopped

2 stalks scallions, white and light green parts only, sliced

½ jalapeño, sliced (optional)

Preparation

Heat oil in a medium stockpot over medium-high heat. Cook onions, garlic, ginger, and red pepper flakes just until the onions turn translucent, about 4 minutes.

Add the chicken broth, coconut milk, lime zest, and fish sauce. Bring to a boil. Lower to a simmer and add the sliced mushrooms, cook for 5 minutes. Season to taste.

Meanwhile, soak and drain the rice noodles according to package instructions.

Bring the soup back up to a boil, and add the sliced chicken. Cook until the chicken is no longer pink, about 5 minutes. Stir in the spinach and cook for 2 minutes.

Turn off the heat and stir in the lime juice, cilantro leaves, and scallions.

Divide the rice noodles between 4 bowls. Pour the hot broth over the noodles. Serve with jalapeño slices, if using.

Basic Miso Soup

Ingredients

3 cups water

1 3-inch piece of kombu (dried kelp)

2 tablespoons miso shiro paste (white miso; see Chef Tips)

2 tablespoons sliced scallions (optional)

Preparation

In a medium saucepan bring the water and kombu to a boil. Turn heat down to low and remove kombu, dry and reserve for another use. Transfer ½ cup of broth to a small bowl, and whisk with miso paste until well blended.

Turn off the heat, and return the miso mixture to the saucepan. Stir well and serve with scallion, if using.

Chicken & Rice Soup

Ingredients

1 teaspoon olive oil

½ medium onion, chopped

4 celery ribs, diced

3 medium carrots, diced

2 teaspoons dill, fresh or dried

½ cup long-grain brown rice (or white rice, see Chef Tips)

Salt and pepper, to taste

2 pounds chicken breast on the bone, skinned

5 cups water (or broth)

Chopped parsley, to garnish (optional)

Preparation

Heat the olive oil in a large pot over medium heat. Add the onions, celery, carrots, dill, rice, salt, and pepper. Cook, stirring occasionally, until the vegetables are tender and the onions are translucent, about 8 minutes.

Add the chicken and 4 cups of water. Bring to a boil, then cover and simmer for 1 hour, adding more water if too much evaporates.

Remove the chicken and transfer to a colander. Once cool enough to handle, shred the chicken meat off the bone and return to the broth to heat through. Discard the bones. Taste the soup for seasonings, add parsley if using, and serve.

Yogurt Marinade

Ingredients

1 cup plain yogurt

1 medium shallot, minced

3 tablespoons olive oil

1 tablespoon lemon juice

½ teaspoon lemon zest

½ teaspoon garam marsala

1 tablespoon chopped cilantro

Preparation

Blend all the marinade ingredients together until smooth. Use immediately, or store in the fridge for up to 3 days.

Pumpkin Miso Soup

Ingredients

1 small kabocha pumpkin, washed, halved, and seeds scraped out

2 tablespoon grapeseed or canola oil

1 large Spanish onion, thinly sliced

8 to 10 cups low-sodium stock or water

2 to 3 tablespoons yellow miso paste (miso shiro), or to taste

Sea salt and black pepper, to taste

Soy sauce (optional)

Preparation

With a peeler, take off little patches of skin all over the pumpkin halves until they look polka dotted. This is purely decorative and can be left out if you don't have time. Cut the halves into a ½-inch dice. Set aside.

Heat the oil in a large soup pot over a medium-high heat. When it ripples, add the onion and saute, stirring until the onion starts to soften and turn transparent. Add the pumpkin cubes, sprinkle with a little sea salt, mix well, and cover. Turn the heat down to medium low and sweat the vegetables for about 10 minutes, or until the pumpkin has started to soften and the onion is soft. The onion should not brown, so stir the pot occasionally to make sure it doesn't stick.

Add enough stock to the pot to cover the vegetables plus 1 inch. Raise the heat and bring to a boil. Cover, turn the heat to low, and simmer until the pumpkin is soft but not mushy, about 10 minutes. Do not overcook! While the soup is cooking, measure the miso into a bowl. Using a small balloon whisk or a fork, gradually whisk in ½ cup of warm stock or cool water until you have a thinnish, creamy-looking liquid with no lumps.

When the pumpkin is tender, add a grind or two of black pepper and turn off the heat. Add the miso cream little by little, stirring gently to mix. Taste as you go until you know how much you like. Miso is richly salty, so you do not want too much in the soup. Check for seasoning. Serve immediately.

Gingersnap Peach Crunch

Ingredients

4 pounds peaches, peeled, pitted and sliced*

1/4 cup plus 2 Tablespoons dark brown sugar

2 Tablespoons fresh lemon juice

2 Tablespoons unsalted butter

1/4 cup plus 2 Tablespoons flour

pinch salt

1 cup coarsely crushed gingersnaps (used 60 Trader Joe's Lowfat Ginger Cat Cookies for people)

Preparation

Preheat oven to 400 degrees. Spray a non-stick skillet with cooking spray. Add peaches and cook over high heat until softened (about 10 minutes).

Add 1/4 cup dark brown sugar and lemon juice and cook until juices get thick and syrupy and peaches are soft (approximately 5 minutes). Pour into a 10" deep dish pie plate or 1 1/2 – 2 quart baking dish.

Meanwhile, pulse butter, flour, salt and remaining dark brown sugar in a food processor until the mixture resembles coarse meal. Add the gingersnaps and pulse just to incorporate.

Press the topping into clump and sprinkle over peaches. Bake 15-20 minutes until the top is browned and the filling is bubbly.

Do Less Day Marinated Roasted Wild Salmon

Ingredients

16 ounce wild Coho (Silver) salmon fillet*

Marinade:

thumb sized piece of fresh ginger, peeled and grated

2 cloves garlic, germ removed, peeled and grated

splash Ponzu Sauce (or Soy Sauce)-Ponzu is a citrus infused soy sauce.

1 tablespoon frozen orange juice concentrate

splash dry French white vermouth

Topping:

1 tablespoon dark brown sugar

salt and pepper

Preparation

Combine marinade ingredients, pour over salmon and marinate for about an hour. Preheat oven to 400 degrees. Remove salmon from marinade and place in a baking dish. Sprinkle with dark brown sugar, salt and pepper. Roast until just cooked through-approximately 15 minutes.

Pear & Peach Sorbet

Ingredients

2 15-16 ounce cans pear or peach halves in heavy syrup

Direction

Freeze unopened cans of fruit for a minimum of 8 hours. Dip unopened cans in hot water for 20 seconds to loosen filling. Pour contents into the bowl of a food processor (I used my Vitamix) tearing at the filling with a fork to break up the pieces of fruit. Puree until smooth. Transfer sorbet to a covered container and refreeze. When ready to serve, remove from the freezer and let soften for approximately 5 minutes.

New Breakfast Smoothie (Kefir Berry Protein Smoothie)

Ingredients

1/2 cup plain low fat or non fat Kefir*

1/2 frozen banana

1/3 cup frozen blueberries (wild usually)

handful frozen strawberries (about 4 large berries)

1 scoop unflavored whey protein isolate**

1 tablespoon almond butter

Preparation

Puree until smooth and there are no flecks.

Note: Kefir is cultured milk and is also considered a "fermented" food. I use Lifeway Kefir without added fiber. It has a sour, cultured taste that is stronger than yogurt. It also contains 10 probiotic strains and 11 grams of protein per cup.

Protein Powered Onion Soup Dip

Ingredients

1 6 ounce cup fat free Greek yogurt

2 teaspoons onion powder (or more depending on taste)

1 teaspoon Better Than Gravy gravy mix for beef (sold in a 1 ounce envelope)

freshly ground black pepper

finely snipped chives (optional)

Preparation

Combine all ingredients and stir until smooth. Enjoy with baked chips of your choice. Pictured above with Kettle Brand Baked Chips sea salt flavor.

Low-fat Lemon Buttermilk Tea Bread

Ingredients

1 3/4 cups flour

3/4 cups sugar

2 teaspoons baking powder

1/4 teaspoon salt

1 egg

1 cup buttermilk

1/4 cup canola oil

2 teaspoons finely grate lemon peel

3 tablespoons lemon juice

1 tablespoon sugar

Preparation

Preheat oven to 350 degrees. Spray the bottom and sides of a 9×5 inch pan and line the bottom with parchment paper. Mix flour, 3/4 cup sugar, baking powder and salt in a medium bowl. In another bowl mix egg, buttermilk, oil, lemon peel and 1 tablespoon of lemon juice until well blended. Add buttermilk mixture to flour mixture and stir until just moistened (there may be some lumps). Spread mixture in prepared pan.

Bake 50-60 minutes or until golden brown and a toothpick inserted in the center comes out clean. Meanwhile, mix remaining lemon juice with 1 tablespoon of sugar. Brush mixture over the top of the warm bread then cool in the pan on a rack for 10 minutes, remove bread from pan and cool an additional hour. When completely cool, wrap in plastic wrap. This bread is best served the next day.

Frozen Banana Peanut Butter Chocolate Chip Milkshake

Ingredients

1/2 cup unsweetened vanilla almond milk

1 tablespoon peanut butter (Trader Joe's Creamy Salted-just salt and peanuts)

1 frozen banana*

1 square Lindt 85% Extra Dark chocolate**

Direction

Place all ingredients into a blender and puree until smooth and creamy.

Squash Herb Bread

Things To Get

1 1/2 cups roasted, mashed butternut squash (I used canned pumpkin)

2 cups flour

2 teaspoons baking powder

1/2 teaspoon salt

1 teaspoon herb seasoning (I used Italian Herb Mix)

2 tablespoons olive oil

1/4 cup cold water

Direction

Preheat oven to 400 degrees. Combine ingredients with a large spoon in a large bowl. Place on a lightly floured surface and knead until soft and spongy adding a little more flour if the dough is too sticky. Do not over knead. Form into a round loaf approximately 6 inches in diameter. Place on a parchment lined baking sheet and cut a cross in the top with a sharp knife that has been dipped in flour. Bake for 35-40 minutes. Remove loaf with oven mitts and carefully tap the bottom. It should sound hollow. If it doesn't, return the bread to the oven for an additional 5 minutes. Cut into wedges and enjoy.

Spring Pea & Lettuce Soup

Ingredients

2 teaspoons extra virgin olive oil

1 medium onion, chopped

1 clove garlic, chopped

1 head Romaine lettuce (approximately 1 pound) including dark green outer leaves, washed, trimmed and thinly sliced

10 ounces frozen baby peas, rinsed

1 cup low sodium chicken broth

1 1/2 cups water

3/4 teaspoon salt

pepper, to taste

1 tablespoon finely chopped fresh dill

fresh lemon juice

Preparation

Spray the interior of a large soup pot with cooking spray, add olive oil and saute onion until soft (approximately 5 minutes). Add garlic and saute an additional minute. Stir in lettuce and cook until wilted (approximately 3 minutes). Add peas, broth, water, salt and pepper. Bring to a boil and simmer uncovered for 10 minutes. The lettuce should be very wilted and the peas should look "puckered". Stir in dill during the last minute of cooking. Puree thoroughly then press through a fine, mesh strainer before returning to the pot.

Adjust seasoning with salt and pepper. Season each serving with a squeeze of fresh lemon.

Impromptu Sweet Potato and Butternut Squash Soup

Ingredients

1 sweet potato (any size), peeled and cubed

2 cups (or so) roasted butternut squash (or equivalent frozen puree or cubes)

low sodium chicken stock

palmful of onion powder

1 garlic clove (less or more depending on your taste), grated

1 cube Ginger Paste

pinch thyme leaves

2 canned pear halves

palmful pumpkin pie spice

palmful mild curry powder

2 glugs maple syrup (I like Grade B)

salt and pepper to taste

Preparation

Bring sweet potato cubes and enough chicken stock to cover to a boil. Reduce heat and add remaining ingredients except curry powder. Simmer until sweet potato cubes are very tender. Puree and return to the soup pot. Thin to desired consistency with stock. Season with curry powder and salt and pepper to taste.

Impromptu Carrot Ginger Soup

Ingredients

carrots, peeled and chopped

low sodium chicken stock

palmful of onion powder

1 garlic clove (less or more depending on taste) grated

1 cube Ginger Paste

pinch of curry powder or pumpkin pie spice

salt and pepper to taste

Preparation

Bring all ingredients (except curry powder) to a boil in enough chicken stock to cover. Simmer until very tender. Puree and return to soup pot. Thin to desired consistency with stock. Season with curry powder or pumpkin pie spice, salt and pepper.

Baked Potato Tuna Salad

Ingredients

Serves 1

1/2 leftover baked potato, skin removed and cubed (approximately 6 ounces)

1/2 of a 5 ounce can of white tuna in water, drained

1 tablespoon mayo of your choice (I like Hellman's Olive Oil Mayo)

fresh lemon juice

onion powder to taste

salt free seasoning-I like Penzey's Mural of Flavor (optional)

salt and pepper

Direction

Combine ingredients and season to taste.

Asparagus Soup

Ingredients

1 teaspoon olive oil

1 shallot, chopped

1 pound of asparagus, trimmed and chopped-tips reserved

4 cups low sodium chicken stock

salt and pepper to taste

Preparation

Spray a soup pot with cooking spray. When pot is hot add olive oil and shallot. Salt lightly and saute the shallot until tender and starting to turn golden. Add asparagus pieces (reserving the tips) and saute for a minute or so. Add chicken stock and bring to a boil. Simmer UNCOVERED (to preserve the beautiful green color) until asparagus is very tender. Puree thoroughly and press through a fine mesh sieve to catch any stringy fibers. Return soup to the pot and adjust seasoning with salt and pepper.

Meanwhile, bring a small pot of water to a boil, salt the water then drop the asparagus tips in. Cook until very tender. DO NOT cover or the asparagus will lose its beautiful green color. Time will depend on how big the tips are. When tender drain and shock in a small bowl of ice water to stop cooking.

Serve each cup of soup with a garnish of asparagus tips.

Quickie Salmon and Corn Chowder

Ingredients

3 ounces cooked salmon, flaked

1 4 ounce jar Earth's Best Organic Corn and Butternut Squash baby food

1/2 cup fat free milk (or milk substitute) I just filled the empty baby food jar

generous sprinkling of Penzey's Mural of Flavor salt free seasoning

salt and pepper (be generous as baby food is under-seasoned)

pinch Spanish smoked paprika (optional)

Preparation

Combine all ingredients in a saucepan and simmer until warmed through

Melon Green Smoothie

Ingredient

1 cup mixed melon balls

1/2 handful baby spinach

Juice from 1/2 a lime

1 scoop of vanilla protein

Preparation

Blend and enjoy.

Choc Dream Smoothie

Ingredients

1/2- 1 frozen banana

1/4 cup frozen zucchini

1/4 cup frozen avocado

1 handful baby spinach

1 tbsp nut butter of choice (I prefer almond butter or cashew butter)

1 cup almond milk

1 scoop chocolate protein

1 tbsp chocolate magnesium (optional)

1 tsp trace minerals (optional)

Direction

Blend & enjoy! This smoothie provides lots of great fats that are easy to digest, which normally, Gastroparesis patients have a hard time digesting. Plus, the cacao offers a ton of magnesium, which is great for the muscles.

Berry Blast Smoothie

Ingredients

1 cup mixed berries or just strawberries

1/4 handful baby spinach

1 cup coconut milk

1 scoop vanilla protein

Preparation

Blend & enjoy!

Easy Green Smoothie

Ingredients

1/2 cup frozen pineapple chunks

1/4 cup frozen zucchini

1 handful baby spinach

Juice from 1 lime

1 cup coconut water

1 scoop vanilla protein of choice (optional, but highly recommend)

1 tsp trace minerals (optional but highly recommend)

Preparation

Blend and enjoy.

Note: This smoothie is great to provide a TON of greens and the vitamins and minerals needed without it being too hard to digest. I highly recommend the trace minerals because more than likely, you are severely lacking most of the minerals your body needs, and this will provide that in an easy-to-absorb way. Do not overdo the drops, because it will taste like metal.

Chapter 7: Final Thought

Gastroparesis presents a multifaceted challenge for patients, caregivers, and healthcare providers alike. This complex condition, characterized by delayed stomach emptying, can significantly impact quality of life and pose various health risks if left unmanaged. Throughout this book, we have delved into the intricacies of gastroparesis, exploring its causes, symptoms, diagnosis, and treatment options.

While managing gastroparesis can be daunting, there is hope and empowerment in understanding the condition and its management strategies. From dietary modifications and lifestyle adjustments to medical interventions and emotional support, individuals living with gastroparesis have a range of tools at their disposal to navigate the challenges posed by this condition.

Moreover, ongoing research and advancements in medical science offer promise for improved outcomes and better quality of life for gastroparesis patients in the future. By staying informed, proactive, and connected to supportive networks, individuals affected by gastroparesis can better cope with its challenges and strive for a fulfilling life despite its limitations.

As we close this chapter on gastroparesis, let us remember the importance of compassion, resilience, and advocacy in supporting those affected by this condition. By working together, we can enhance awareness, promote research, and ultimately improve the lives of individuals living with gastroparesis.

Dietary Advice

When managing gastroparesis, it's essential to be mindful of both the frequency and sequence of your meals. Healthcare professionals often recommend consuming five to eight small meals throughout the day to facilitate digestion and minimize discomfort. Additionally, thorough chewing before swallowing can aid in the digestive process and reduce the strain on your stomach.

To optimize nutrition intake and prevent feeling overly full from meals that may not provide sufficient nourishment, prioritize consuming nutrient-dense foods at the beginning of each meal. This approach ensures that your body receives essential nutrients before you feel full, helping to maintain a balanced diet despite the challenges posed by gastroparesis.

Considering the potential nutritional deficiencies associated with gastroparesis, incorporating a multivitamin supplement into your daily routine can help bridge the gap and ensure that you're meeting your body's requirements for essential vitamins and minerals. Especially during the recovery phase, when nutrient absorption may be compromised, a multivitamin supplement can provide valuable support for overall health and well-being.

If weight loss has been a concern due to gastroparesis-related symptoms, it's important to prioritize calorie intake to support your body's energy needs and promote recovery. Starting with a minimum daily calorie intake of 1,500 calories can help prevent further weight loss and provide the energy necessary for healing and rehabilitation.

In addition to solid foods, nutritional beverages can play a crucial role in meeting your dietary needs while managing gastroparesis. These liquid options are easy to digest and can help supplement your nutrient intake, particularly when solid foods may be challenging to tolerate. Examples of nutritional beverages include smoothies made with yogurt or a combination of fruits and vegetables, which provide a convenient and nutritious option for individuals with gastroparesis.

Protein shakes are another valuable option for individuals struggling to meet their protein needs through traditional meals. These liquid meal replacement shakes offer a concentrated source of protein and essential nutrients, making them an excellent choice for maintaining muscle mass and supporting overall health during gastroparesis recovery.

By carefully considering your dietary choices, incorporating nutrient-rich foods and beverages, and ensuring adequate calorie and protein intake, you can support your body's nutritional needs while managing the challenges of gastroparesis. Working closely with healthcare professionals, including dietitians and gastroenterologists, can provide personalized guidance and support to help you navigate the complexities of dietary management in gastroparesis effectively.

Nutritional Recommendation

Ensuring adequate hydration is paramount for maintaining optimal digestive health. Hydration supports the smooth movement of food through the digestive tract, aiding in the prevention of constipation and promoting overall gastrointestinal function. Therefore, it is advisable to consume plenty of water, especially for individuals experiencing symptoms of gastroparesis.

Conversely, alcohol consumption should be limited or avoided altogether for individuals with gastroparesis symptoms. Alcohol has a dehydrating effect on the body, which can exacerbate symptoms of dehydration and constipation. Moreover, alcohol consumption may deplete essential nutrients from the body, further compromising overall health and well-being.

Gastroparesis, while often a chronic condition, can sometimes present acutely, indicating underlying health concerns or occurring without a clear cause. Regardless of the duration or underlying cause of gastroparesis, dietary adjustments play a crucial role in symptom management and overall well-being. Eating smaller, more frequent meals and reducing intake of high-fiber and high-fat foods can facilitate digestion and alleviate discomfort associated with gastroparesis.

Individuals with gastroparesis may find that certain foods are better tolerated than others, depending on their specific diagnosis and individual tolerances. Consulting with a healthcare professional or a registered dietitian is essential for developing a personalized nutrition plan tailored to individual needs and preferences. It is imperative to ensure that the body continues to receive adequate vitamins and minerals necessary for optimal organ function as one navigates through the challenges of managing gastroparesis symptoms.

Although gastroparesis is a chronic illness with no known cure, it is manageable through various approaches, including dietary modifications, medication management, and proper blood glucose control. While adjustments may be necessary, individuals with gastroparesis can still lead fulfilling lives by prioritizing self-care, seeking appropriate medical guidance, and making informed lifestyle choices. With proper management and support, individuals with gastroparesis can achieve improved symptom control and maintain overall health and wellness.

www.ingramcontent.com/pod-product-compliance
Lightning Source LLC
Chambersburg PA
CBHW050201230526
45470CB00001B/188